Equalities and Inequalities in Health

Equalities and Inequalities in Health

Proceedings of the Twelfth Annual Symposium of the Eugenics Society London 1975

Edited by

C. O. CARTER

Institute of Child Health, London

JOHN PEEL

Teesside Polytechnic, Middlesbrough, Teesside

1976

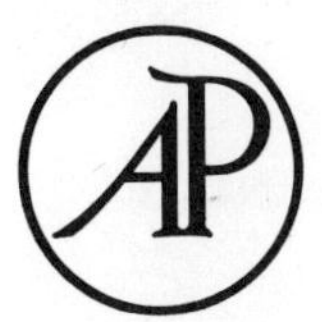

Academic Press

London · New York · San Francisco

A Subsidiary of Harcourt Brace Jovanovich, Publishers,

ACADEMIC PRESS INC. (LONDON) LTD.
24/28 Oval Road,
London, NW1

United States Edition published by
ACADEMIC PRESS INC.
111 Fifth Avenue
New York, New York 10003

Library of Congress Catalog Card Number 0–12–161850–1
ISBN: 76–016957

SET IN GREAT BRITAIN BY GLOUCESTER TYPESETTING CO. LTD., GLOUCESTER,
PRINTED BY J. W. ARROWSMITH LTD., BRISTOL

Contributors

MILDRED BLAXTER, *Institute of Medical Sociology, Westburn Road, Aberdeen AB9 2ZE, Scotland*

SIR JOHN BROTHERSTON, *Scottish Home and Health Department, St Andrew's House, Edinburgh EH1 3DE, Scotland*

C. O. CARTER, *MRC Clinical Genetics Unit, Institute of Child Health, 30 Guilford Street, London WC1N 1EH, England*

R. J. DONALDSON, *Centre for Extension Training in Community Medicine, 31 Bedford Square, London WC1B 3EL, England*

J. H. EDWARDS, *The Infant Development Unit, Queen Elizabeth Medical Centre, Edgbaston, Birmingham B15 2TG, England*

DONALD GOULD, *Medical Correspondent,* New Statesman, *10 Great Turnstile Street, London WC1V 7HJ, England*

G. MELVYN HOWE, *Department of Geography, University of Strathclyde, 26 Richmond Street, Glasgow G1 1XH, Scotland*

P. J. HUNTINGFORD, *Department of Obstetrics and Gynaecology, The London Hospital Medical College, Turner Street, London E1 2AD England*

W. R. LEE, *Department of Occupational Health, University of Manchester, Oxford Road, Manchester M13 9PT, England*

D. M. POTTS, *Population Services International, 500 Chesham House, 150 Regent Street, London W1, England*

D. M. PRINSLEY, *Department of Geriatric Medicine, Poole Hospital, Middlesbrough, Cleveland TS7 0NH, England*

D. F. ROBERTS, *Department of Human Genetics, University of Newcastle upon Tyne NE2 4AA, England*

Preface

This volume contains the texts of papers presented at the twelfth annual Symposium of the Eugenics Society held in September 1975. It is the second in a trilogy devoted to equalities and inequalities in contemporary society, the first having been concerned with education.

The recent history of advanced industrial societies has shown that the demand for health care services, as for education, is virtually insatiable and that health facilities, like educational provision, are regarded as self-evidently desirable.

The Eugenics Society, having a traditional concern with all those factors contributing to the quality of life, felt it opportune to review, in this Symposium, our present knowledge of the contributions made by medicine to human welfare. We are grateful to the distinguished contributors, who represent a wide variety of disciplines, for their willingness to speak to guidelines suggested by the editors.

The editors, once again, acknowledge with thanks the help given by Miss Eileen Walters in the detailed organization of this Symposium; also that of Mrs Mavis Warnes who typed the final draft of the papers.

On behalf of the Eugenics Society
C. O. Carter
John Peel

September 1976

Contents

The Global Incidence of Genetic Disease

C. O. CARTER
Medical Research Council Clinical Genetics Unit, Institute of Child Health, London, England

Introduction

In this review I will discuss the frequency at birth of genetic disorders in Britain, the country for which we have on the whole the best data, and discuss some evidence for different frequencies in other parts of the world and other racial groups.

I should define birth frequency and genetic disease.

BIRTH FREQUENCY

The epidemiologist is concerned with the "prevalence" of disease, by which he usually means the proportion of the whole population who have a disease at a particular point in time. He may also speak of the prevalence in a particular age group, for example adolescents or the new-born. The geneticist is usually more interested in the proportion of the population at birth who have the genetic abnormality even though in some cases, for example Huntington's chorea, they will not develop the clinical disease till many years later. This is the sense in which I am using birth frequency. Again congenital malformations are by definition present at birth, but if the patients have only a short life-span the prevalence of congenital malformations will fall off sharply with increasing age and their prevalence in the whole population will be relatively low. Patients with Down's syndrome (mongolism) have a frequency in Britain of about one in 700 live births, but by age 10 the prevalence is about one in 1,000 and the prevalence at age 40 years is low. Patients with Huntington's chorea have been found in surveys in different areas of Britain, Canada and Australia to have an overall prevalence of one in 10,000 to one in 20,000. The onset of the disease may be as early as

10 years or as later as 70 years, but is usually between 30 and 50 years. The usual duration of the disorder from onset till death is some 10 to 15 years. This is about one sixth of the usual expectation of life. One may estimate then that the birth frequency of those who carry the dominant mutant gene responsible for Huntington's chorea is about six times higher than the prevalence, that is about one in 2,000. This is the number who will at some time develop the disease if they live to 70.

GENETIC DISEASE

There are three main forms of genetic predisposition to malformation and disease: chromosome abnormalities; mutant genes of large effect occurring at a single gene locus; polygenic determination, by which it is implied that the genetic predisposition depends on the accumulation of relatively minor genetic variation at several, perhaps many gene loci. With the latter type of genetic causation there is usually also interaction with the environment.

The birth frequency of conditions due to chromosomal anomalies probably varies little between different countries and different races. The birth frequency of monogenic conditions, that is those due to mutant genes of large effect, probably varies little when the disease is dominant, but may vary widely when the disease is recessive. The birth frequency of polygenically determined disorders may also show wide geographical and racial variation.

Chromosal Anomalies

The birth frequency of patients with chromosomal anomalies causing clinical disorder among live births is fairly accurately known, at least for those readily recognized microscopically. The total load is about four per 1,000 live births. The birth frequency of the most common severe anomaly of this kind, trisomy 21, responsible for Down's syndrome, was established some years ago by careful clinical examination of the new-born (Carter and McCarthy, 1951). This has been confirmed and the frequency of other chromosomal anomalies established by several large series in which all new-born babies have been screened by making chromosome preparations from a drop of blood (Jacobs *et al*, 1974). In this way it is not difficult to pick up the presence of extra or missing chromosomes, or large parts of chromosomes. Recently new staining techniques have been developed which show up light and dark bands on the chromosomes and enable small chromosome changes to be detected, but these have not yet been applied in routine screening surveys.

The total load of four per 1,000 live births with major chromosome anomalies is about equally divided into abnormality of sex-chromosome pair and abnormalities of the other 22 pairs, which are collectively called "autosomes". The relatively high frequency of abnormalities of the sex-chromosome pair is due to the fact that most of the autosomal anomalies present at conception cause the death of the fetus and spontaneous abortion in the first three months of pregnancy. About 40 per cent of first three month spontaneous abortions are found to be due to a major autosomal anomaly.

The breakdown of the 2·0 per 1,000 autosomal anomalies among live births is summarized in Table I.

TABLE I

Frequency of unbalanced autosomal anomalies per 1,000 live births

Trisomy 21 (Down's syndrome)	1·5
Trisomy 18 (Edwards' syndrome)	0·1
Trisomy 13 (Patau's syndrome)	0·1
Miscellaneous (mainly structural)	0·3
Total	2·0

Trisomy 21, 18 and 13 all cause syndromes clinically recognizable at birth. The abnormalities caused by trisomy 18 and 13 are however so serious that the child rarely survives infancy. Down's anomaly on the other hand though associated with an increased mortality at all ages, but especially in the first year, is compatible in some instances with survival to age 70 years. This single condition is responsible now for about a third of all cases of severe mental retardation at primary school age. It is noteworthy that even with trisomy 21 the frequency at conception is at least twice as high as among live births. It is also noteworthy that probably no fetuses with a missing autosome survive the first few weeks of fetal life. In addition about two per 1,000 babies are born with a balanced chromosomal anomaly which will cause no clinical disturbance but may predispose them to have chromosomally abnormal children.

The breakdown of the 2·0 per 1,000 sex-chromosomal anomalies is summarized in Table II. The normal male sex chromosome pair consists of a X and Y, written XY, and the normal female sex pair consists of two Xs, and is written XX.

The sex-chromosomal trisomies XYY, XXY, and XXX do not appear to result in an increased liability to abort and hence their high frequency

TABLE II

Frequency of sex-chromosomal anomalies per 1,000 live births

(a) Boys	
XYY (extra Y syndrome)	1·0
XXY (Klinefelter syndrome)	1·0
(b) Girls	
XXX (triple X syndrome)	1·0
Both sexes	
Miscellaneous	0·5
Total both sexes	2·0

among live-born. In contrast at least 95 per cent of the fetuses with just a single X chromosome, written XO, spontaneously abort. Even the five per cent survival is remarkable since as I noted above a complete missing autosome probably invariably causes early abortion. The explanation of the relatively lesser effects of extra or missing X chromosomes is that early in fetal life any X chromosome above one becomes inactive, and so after about three weeks of fetal life an XXY male is effectively an XY male, and an XXX female as well as a normal XX female effectively has a single X operative. Tolerance of an extra Y chromosome probably depends on the fact that this chromosome appears to carry only masculinizing genes or indeed perhaps one single masculinizing gene. The clinical effects of the trisomies are therefore not dramatic. However both XXY and XXX trisomies appear to shift the distribution of intelligence quotient about 10 points to the left, so that they are relatively frequent among the mentally retarded. The XYYs tend to be tall, with a mean height of about six feet instead of five feet eight inches, to have dense bones and probably an undue amount of male impulsiveness and aggression. They are fertile. The XXY males have small testes, are infertile and often have a eunuchoid physique. The XXX females are on the whole normal though they are sub-fertile and have menstrual irregularities. The XO girls at birth have a number of physical stigmata such as short stature and neck webbing but also are sterile with ovaries at birth replaced by fibrous streaks and hence no spontaneous secondary sex development, but are normally intelligent.

It is noteworthy that both the autosomal trisomies and the XXY and XXX forms of sex-chromosomal trisomies occur with increasing frequency with increasing maternal age. This has long been known for Down's syndrome where the birth frequency rises from about one in 2,000 for mother's age 20–25, to over one in 100 for mothers over the age of 40. There is no effect of paternal age.

Geographical varition: the non-disjunction of chromosome pairs is the formation of sperm and ova, responsible for the formation of trisomies and monosomies appears to be a biological accident which occurs widely in mammals and indeed even in plants. Down's syndrome has been suspected clinically and demonstrated microscopically in a baby chimpanzee, now unfortunately dead. Chromosomal non-disjunction probably occurs with much the same frequency in man all over the world, when allowance is made for different distributions of maternal age.

Conditions Due to Mutant Genes of Large Effect

It is much more difficult to estimate the total birth frequency in a population of babies with monogenic determination of serious disease. In contrast to the non-disjunction of chromosome pairs, gene mutations are individually rare events. There are however very many gene loci and so while individual monogenic conditions if clinically serious tend to be rare, there are many hundreds of such conditions already recognized, more are being recognized every year. The total birth frequency is perhaps twice as high as that of conditions due to chromosomal anomalies and of the order of 10 per 1,000 live births. The information available consists mostly of careful surveys of individual monogenic conditions in particular populations. Naturally enough it is the more common conditions which have been surveyed in this way and the birth frequencies found from them are almost certainly unrepresentative of most monogenic conditions.

Monogenically determined conditions are conveniently divided into dominant, recessive and X-linked. Dominant conditions in medical terminology are those in which patients have only a single dose of the mutant gene. In the 1975 catalogue of monogenically determined disorders compiled by Professor McKusick of Baltimore, 583 conditions are listed as dominant with another 635 listed as possibly dominant. Some of these are of only minor effect and may be regarded almost as normal variants. Some are extremely rare, but the experienced medical geneticist will have seen most of them at one time or another in the course of his daily work. Estimates of birth frequencies for some of the dominant conditions from which surveys have been made are shown in Table III.

For reasons given above these must not be taken as typical of severe or moderately severe dominant conditions, most of which probably have a frequency at birth of 0·01 to 0·001 per 1,000. Where a dominant condition has an early onset and is sufficiently severe to prevent reproduction almost all cases will be due to fresh mutations and the birth frequency will be double the mutation rate (double because mutation

TABLE III

Birth frequencies of some more common dominant conditions in European derived populations per 1000 live births

Nervous system	
Huntington's chorea	0·5 (Shokeir, 1975)
Neurofibromatosis	0·4 (Crowe *et al.*, 1956)
Myotonic dystrophy	0·2 (Grimm, 1975; Klein, 1958)
Intestines	
Multiple polyposis coli	0·1 (Veale, 1965; Reed and Reed, 1958)
Kidney	
Polycystic disease of the kidneys	0·8 (Dalgaard, 1957)
Locomotor system	
Diaphyseal aclasia	0·5 (Murken, 1963)
Sight	
Dominant forms of blindness	0·1 (Fraser and Friedmann, 1967)
Hearing	
Dominant forms of deafness	0·1 (Stevenson and Cheeseman, 1955; Chung *et al.*, 1958)

rates are given per germ cell, sperm or ovum, and not per fertilized egg-cell). The relatively high frequency of a condition such as Huntington's chorea is because the onset of the disease is often after the patient has already had children. The mutant gene may then be passed down and affect individuals in several generations. Multiple polyposes of the colon may not become malignant and so cause death till the 30s or 40s. A recently recognized monogenic disorder, monogenic familial hypercholesterolaemia, which causes the death from ischaemic heart disease of about half the men affected by age 60 years, may have a birth frequency of about two in 1,000. The condition may well have been less dangerous in earlier populations who took more exercise and ate less fat.

As with conditions due to chromosomal anomalies the limited information indicates that some dominant conditions have much the same frequency in all races of man. Gene mutation is again a basic biological accident. For some such conditions variation in the distribution of paternal age may have an effect since the frequency of some dominant mutations increases with increasing paternal age, though the influence is not as strong as the maternal age effect in trisomies. Less severe dominant conditions may show variation in frequency, especially in small populations or populations which have grown rapidly from originally small numbers as a result of chance-founder effect and drift. A well known example is the high frequency of porphyria in South Africans of Dutch descent which may be traced back to the progeny of a single emigrant from Holland. It caused little trouble until the introduction of barbiturate drugs, but the ingestion of these may kill those who have the condition.

Recessive conditions in medical terminology are those in which affected individuals have a double dose of the mutant gene concerned. Both parents happen to carry a single dose of the mutant gene concerned but are themselves unaffected by it, whereas if the mutant gene had been dominant such individuals would be clinically abnormal. The chance of any individual child receiving the mutant gene from both his carrier parents is one in four. In general recessive conditions are, understandably, more severe than dominants at least until recently when patients rarely survived to have children. There is however no selection against the mutant gene in the carrier and so such mutant genes may be transmitted for many generations, over hundreds or even thousands of years before they meet another mutant gene of the same kind in a particular patient. This is more likely to happen where a married couple are blood-relatives, for example first cousins. Because of the long gap between the mutational event and the occurrence of a patient there is the opportunity for several influences to affect the birth frequency of recessive conditions: chance founder effect and drift, changes in the frequency of consanguineous marriage and in a few exceptional instances an actual selective advantage of those who carry the mutant gene, in single dose, even though a double dose is lethal.

The number of conditions listed in McKusick's catalogue as certainly or very likely recessive is 466 with 481 possibly recessive. Once again this includes some minor conditions and some very rare ones, but mostly conditions that the experienced medical geneticist will see at some time in his working life.

The birth frequency of some of the more common recessive conditions in Britain is shown in Table IV.

The recessive condition whose frequency is outstandingly high is cystic fibrosis a condition which usually causes death in childhood from intestinal obstruction or recurrent bronchopheumonia. The figure shown in Table IV is based on prevalence studies of affected children. Recent studies based on screening of new-born babies in several northwest European cities, including Cardiff and Dublin suggest that the true birth frequency may be as high as one in 1,600. This implies a gene-frequency of the mutant gene of one in 40 and that five per cent of north Europeans carry the gene. This high frequency apparently extends from Ireland, through Germany, Hungary and into European Russia; it probably extends into southern Europe though here surveys are incomplete. Now until recently the condition was almost always lethal in childhood and of the survivors today only the women are

TABLE IV

Birth frequencies of some more common recessive conditions in European derived populations per 1,000 live births

Metabolism	
Cystic fibrosis	0·5 (Hall and Simpkiss, 1968; Wright, 1969)
Phenylketonuria classical	0·1 (Carter, 1973)
Nervous system	
Neurogenic muscle atrophies	0·1 (Pearn, 1973; Pearn and Wilson, 1973)
Red blood cells	
Sickle-cell anaemia	0·1 (Carter, 1973)
Endocrine glands	
Adrenal hyperplasias	0·1 (Hubble, 1966; Rosenbloom and Smith, 1966)
Hearing	
Severe congenital deafness	0·2 (Stevenson and Cheeseman, 1955; Chung, 1958)
Sight	
Recessive forms of blindness	0·4 (Fraser and Friedmann, 1967; Chung, *et al.*, 1958)
Mental retardation severe	
Non-specific recessive forms	0·5 (Carter, personal estimate)

fertile. With such a lethal condition, one would normally expect a birth frequency of the same order as the mutation rate, and even one in 40,000 would be a relatively high mutation rate. In Mongolian and Negro peoples cystic fibrosis probably has a frequency of one in 40,000 or less. It is difficult to visualize such a high frequency arising from founder effect and drift in such a large population as 300 million and the most plausible explanation is that in Europe the carrier has had some selective advantage. Phenylketonuria with a birth frequency of one in 10,000 presents the same problem in less acute form. Once again it appears to be a rare condition in Mongolians and Europeans. Figures for the rest of Europe are coming in from screening programmes and are everywhere high with the highest frequencies, about one in 5,000, in Ireland and also in West Germany. Within Britain there is a cline of increasing frequency as one passes from south-east England to the north and west.

The relative high frequencies for sickle-cell anaemia and thalassaemia represent much higher frequencies, about five per 1,000 in our Negro and eastern Mediterranean immigrants respectively. The sickle-cell anaemia distribution is best understood. The high frequencies are confined essentially to the populations of the areas of West and Central

Africa where there is endemic malignant tertian malaria, and in populations descended therefrom in the United States and the West Indies. The explanation also is well known. Though in Africa patients die in childhood and have a high mortality even in developed countries, the carriers have an advantage in that they are resistant to this severe form of malaria. The parasitized red blood cell of the carrier has a shorter life-span than the parasitized red-cell of an individual who is not a carrier. In consequence the parasite has not the time to complete its necessary life cycle in the red cell and so dies.

The high frequency areas of thalassaemia are more extensive stretching from parts of Italy through Greece, the Near East, parts of Indonesia and into southern China. Once again resistance of the carrier to malaria is the probable explanation, but this has not been proved exclusively.

Mutant genes on the X chromosome are in some degree intermediate in their behaviour between dominant and recessive genes. Since a woman has two homologous X chromosomes, the expression of a mutant gene on one X chromosome may be modified by the expression of the normal gene on the other X chromosome. As mentioned above, there appear to be only masculinizing genes on the Y chromosome and so any mutant gene on a male's single X chromosome will be expressed. Women but not men may carry an X-linked gene without clinical manifestion. The birth frequency of some X-linked conditions is shown in Table V.

TABLE V

Birth frequency of more common X-linked conditions in European derived populations per 1,000 live births

Locomotor system	
Muscle dystrophy—Duchenne	0·2
Blood clotting	
Haemophilia, classical	0·1
Skin	
Ichthyosis	0·1
Mental retardation	
Non-specific X-linked	0·1

Estimates mainly from Stevenson and Kerr, 1967.

Outstanding are the severe form of muscular dystrophy, classical haemophilia, and the as yet recently recognized and not yet well defined X-linked form of mental retardation. But these are not sufficiently high to require any special explanation other than the continuance of the frequency by rather high mutation rates.

On a world-scale only one X-linked condition or rather group of conditions associated with an abnormality of a red-cell enzyme, glucose-6-phosphate dehydrogenase, is unduly frequent. This is responsible for favism in the eastern Mediterranean, a condition in which those affected get some red cell destruction on eating Fava beans, and in another form for the acute red cell destruction in certain Negro peoples when given anti-malarial drugs such as primaquine. The high frequency areas once again are malarious.

Turning now to the disorders for which the genetic predisposition is polygenic, I will discuss among these just the common structural malformations. These are now a major source of stillbirth and infant death. Estimation of the total load depends very much on which malformations are included, but taking only those of at least moderate severity the total load is about 20 per 1,000 total births. The frequency in Britain of the more common of these malformations is shown in Tables VIa and VIb.

Outstanding are the congenital malformations of the heart, with a birth frequency of about six per 1,000 total births and of the central nervous system with a combined frequency of four to five per thousand.

Reasonably accurate figures for the frequency of congenital heart malformations are available only for technically advanced countries, but at present there are no indications of much variation in their frequency in, for example, Sweden and the United States as compared with Britain. Southern Europe and Japan too probably have similar frequencies.

The position is very different for the malformations of the central nervous system which arise essentially from a failure of closure of the neural tube. The neural tube is the embryonic precursor of the brain and spinal cord. If the brain is involved, the malformation is called anencephaly. If the spinal cord is involved, the malformation is called spina bifida cystica. For these two conditions there is a striking cline of increasing frequency within Britain from about three per 1,000 total births in the south-east of the country to up to five per thousand in the Midlands and seven to eight per thousand in the north and west, with the highest frequencies in Ulster. Most other Caucasian populations show values rather less than those in south-east England, but with relatively high frequencies in Egypt and in the Punjab in India. Both Mongolian and Negro populations show low values particularly of spina bifida.

Among the other malformations cleft lip ($\pm$cleft palate) shows a relatively high frequency in Mongolians, an intermediate frequency in Caucasians, and a low frequency in Negroes. Talipes equinovarus, the most severe form of cleft foot is especially common in Polynesians.

TABLE VIa

Congenital malformations having a birth frequency of at least one per 1,000 total births in Britain

Heart	
Malformations, all type	6·0
Central nervous system	
Spina bifida	2·6
Anencephaly	2·0
Intestines	
Pyloric stenosis	3·0
Face	
Cleft lip (±cleft palate)	1·3
Locomotor system	
Dislocation of hip	1·0
Talipes (all types)	1·4
Polydactyly	1·1

Estimates mainly from Leck, *et al.* (1968).

TABLE VIb

Congenital malformations having a birth frequency of between 0.1 and 0.9 per 1,000 total births

Intestines	
Diaphragmatic hernia (not hiatal)	0·5
Atresia of small bowel	0·2
Rectal atresia	0·4
Skeleton	
Webbed fingers and toes	0·7
Mouth	
Cleft palate	0·4
Kidneys	
Renal agenesis	0·4
Cystic kidneys	0·1
Horseshoe kidney	0·1

Estimates mainly from Leck (1968).

The basis of these variations is not established, they are in some degree environmental, for example the large variation in the frequency of central nervous system malformations within Britain is unlikely to be wholly genetic. However the major racial differences, for example between Caucasians and Negroes for central nervous system malformations, are found in many different environments, in West Africa, in the United

States, the West Indies and England, and are probably therefore genetic.

References

Carter, C. O. (1973). Nature and distribution of genetic abnornalities. *J. biosoc. Sci.* **5**, 261.

Carter, C. O. and McCarthy, D. (1951). Incidence of mongolism and its diagnosis in the newborn. *Brit. J. soc. Med.* **5**, 83.

Chung, C. S., Robinson, O. W. and Morton, N. E. (1958). A note on deaf-mutism *Ann. hum. Genet.* **23**, 357.

Crowe, F. W., Schull, W. J. and Neel, J. V. (1956). *A Clinical, Pathological and Genetic Study of Multiple Neurofibromatosis.* Springfield, Illinois: Thomas.

Dalgaard, O. Z. (1957). *Bilateral Polycystic Disease of the Kidneys. Opera ex Domo biol hum hered,* p. 38. Copenhagen: Ejnar Munksgaard.

Fraser, G. R. and Friedmann, A. I. (1967). *The Causes of Blindness in Childhood. A Study of 776 Children with Severe Visual Handicaps.* Baltimore: Johns Hopkins.

Grimm, T. (1975). The age at onset and of death in dystrophia myotonica. *J. Genet. hum.* **23**, 172.

Hall, B. D. and Simpkiss, M. J. (1968). Incidence of cystic fibrosis in Wessex. *J. med. Genet.* **5**, 262.

Hubble, D. (1966). Congenital adrenal hyperplasia. In: *Concepts of Inborn Errors and Defects of Steroid Biosynthesis.* Edited by K. S. Holt and D. W. Raine. Edinburgh: Livingstone.

Jacobs, P. A., Melville, M., Ratcliffe, S., Keay, A. J. and Syme, J. (1974). A cytogenetic study of 11,680 newborn infants. *Ann. hum. Genet.* **37**, 359.

Klein, D. (1958). Le dystrophie myotonique (Steinert) et la myotonie congénitale (Thomsen) en Suisse. *J. Genet. hum.* **7**, (Suppl).

Leck, I., Record, R. G., McKeown, T. and Edwards, J. H. (1968). The incidence of malformations in Birmingham, England 1950–59. *Teratology,* **1**, 263.

Murken, J.-D. (1963). Uber multiple cartilaginäre exostosen. *Z. menschl. Vererb, -u Konstit-Lehre,* **36**, 469.

Pearn, J. H. (1973). The gene frequency of acute Werdnig-Hoffmann disease (SMA type 1). A total population survey in north-east England. *J. med. Genet.* **10**, 260.

Pearn, J. H. and Wilson, J. (1973). Chronic generalised spinal muscular atrophy of infancy and childhood. *Arch. Dis. Childh.* **48**, 768.

Reed, T. E. and Reed, J. V. (1958). A genetic study of multiple polyposis of the colon. *Amer. J. hum. Genet.* **7**, 236.

Rosenbloom, A. L. and Smith, D. W. (1966). Congenital adrenal hyperplasia. *Lancet,* **i**, 660.

Shokeir, M. H. K. (1975). Investigations on Huntington's disease in the Canadian prairies. *Clin. Genet.* **7**, 345.

Stevenson, A. C. and Cheeseman, E. A. (1955). Hereditary deaf-mutism, with particular reference to Northern Ireland. *Ann. hum. Genet.* **10**, 177.

Stevenson, A. C. and Kerr, C. B. (1967). On the distribution of frequencies of mutation to genes determining harmful traits in man. *Mutation Res.* **4**, 339.

Veale, A. M. O. (1965). *Intestinal Polyposis.* London: Cambridge University Press.

Wright, S. W. (1969). *Racial Variations in the Incidence of Cystic Fibrosis.* Proceedings of the Fifth International Conference on Cystic Fibrosis. London: Cystic Fibrosis Research Trust.

Sex Differences in Disease and Mortality

D. F. ROBERTS

Department of Human Genetics, University of Newcastle upon Tyne, England

Sex differences in disease and mortality are but two facets of the multifarious differences in biology that the sex polymorphism confers. Sex is of course determined by the chromosomes of the individual. Omitting from discussion the infrequent intersexes, the normal female karyotype consists of 23 pairs of chromosomes. In the male there are only 22 complete pairs of autosomes, and the 23rd "pair" consists of two dissimilar chromosomes, the X and the Y. Sex depends upon the complement of X and Y chromosomes, and that is determined at the moment of fertilization. If the recipient ovum and the fertilizing sperm both contribute an X chromosome, then the resulting individual will be a female; if either of the combining sex cells contain a Y chromosome, then the resultant individual will be a male.

Although chromosomal sex is determined at conception, it is only at about the eighth week of gestation that the gonadal sex begins to be distinguishable microscopically. By this time the Y chromosome, or rather the masculinizing locus on its short arm, has begun to exert a clear effect on the differentiating cells and their metabolism, for Leydig cells, which secrete testosterone, can be discerned between the medullary cords, so that the male gonad is recognizable as a testis while the female gonad still shows no differentiation. Certainly serum and gonad concentrations of testosterone are already clearly raised in male fetuses by 11–17 weeks (Reyes *et al.*, 1973, 1974). But besides the hormonal stimulation of development of the male organs derived from the Wolffian duct system, the testis secretes another hormone, not an androgen, that suppresses development of female organs from the Mullerian duct system. The fetal testis is a highly active endocrine organ, particularly as regards steroidogenesis, in contrast to the fetal ovary (Challis *et al.*, 1975). But other, related hormones also show clear sex differences. Thus follicular stimulating hormone (FSH) in pituitaries and plasma is higher in females from early in the second trimester. Male differentiation is complete by the fourth month, and thereafter occurs continuation of genital growth and maintenance of function.

Thus fundamental sex differences are established before birth, e.g. in anatomy and morphology, hormonal activity, enzymes, and in skeletal development. Thereafter the sexes continue to diverge as a result of differences in growth patterns and behaviour. At birth boys, on average, are slightly larger than girls, and continue to be so until the girls catch up and temporarily outstrip them by earlier entrance upon the adolescent phase of growth (Tanner, 1962). At this time, the rate of growth increases, with acceleration greater in some dimensions than in others, so that the overall shape of the body changes. The rate of growth of both shoulders and hips increases, but the shoulders grow much more quickly in boys than in girls, so that the shoulder/hip width ratio is quite distinctive.

Similarly, there are changes in body composition (Marshall, 1970). At adolescence, the average boy actually becomes thinner and loses fat, while the average girl continues to put it on, though more slowly during the adolescent spurt than either before or after, so that the body density of boys increases more than that of girls. The growth in muscle in boys is much greater, and so is its acceleration. Muscle strength increases, with quite pronounced differences between the sexes; boys' muscles also become capable of working for longer periods of time, while the amount of oxygen available to them is increased by growth in chest capacity and, in boys, by rapid increase in the number of red blood cells and the amount of haemoglobin in the blood. There is no corresponding rise in girls and indeed there may be a fall. This is particularly clear in populations living near the subsistence level.

Several years ago, with the support of the Eugenics Society, we carried out a survey in Jamaica in a population living close to the subsistence level (Roberts *et al.*, 1966), in the course of which we endeavoured to establish standards for haemoglobin level in normal children there. The haemoglobin levels for boys show a clear trend, increasing with age up to and through adolescence as expected (Table I). In girls, on the other hand, at the younger ages the haemoglobin levels are comparable with those for boys, but the adolescent girls show a significantly lower haemoglobin level both by comparison with the younger girls and with the boys of their own ages, presumably associated with menarche. This perhaps is a point worth remembering, that differences between the

TABLE I

Haemoglobin levels (gr per cent) by age

	Boys		Girls	
Age	Mean	s. d.	Mean	s. d.
1	11·28	1·50		
2	11·51	1·93		
3	11·82	1·27		
4	11·79	1·16		
5	11·52	1·40		
6	12·31	1·32		
7	12·11	1·74	12·24	0·66
8	12·26	1·32	12·43	0·95
9	12·24	1·66	12·39	0·92
10	12·49	0·70	12·36	0·82
11	12·61	1·26	12·36	0·91
12	12·06	0·92	12·30	0·91
13	12·50	1·60	11·74	1·31
14	12·79	1·22	12·01	1·56
15	12·89	1·78	11·78	0·99
16	12·95	0·64		

sexes in biological features may partly depend on the environment and culture in which they live. The most noticeable changes at adolescence are the differences, which are mainly quantitative rather than qualitative, in the development of the secondary sex characters, consequent upon the relatively high output of androgenic hormones in the male and of oestrogen in the female. With the arrival of adulthood the overt cyclic endocrine activity in the female is already well established, in contrast to the continuous level of activity in the male.

Differences in behavioural development accompany body development. Girls learn to talk earlier than boys and then to read earlier, and they also socialize earlier than boys, perhaps because they mature earlier, but also because of a greater interest in people rather than in things or intellectual concepts. These perhaps may be evolutionary preparations for the different adult roles of the two sexes which are found in every society. At the end of reproductive life there occurs relatively suddenly in women the great biological changes associated with the menopause, changes which set them quite apart from the relatively easier male diminution of reproductive activity.

Disease Differences

It is not surprising, therefore, that differences in susceptibility to disease also enter the spectrum of biological sex differences. Sex discrimination is not only a function of society, it is a function of disease. For purposes of discussion we can pick out four types of sex discrimination, overlapping rather than discrete:

conditions primarily or predominantly of genetic origin;
conditions in which environmental factors act unequally on the two sexes;
conditions in which environmental factors might be expected to act equally but in which the incidences are unequal in the two sexes;
conditions directly related to the sex organs.

GENETICS

Monogenic Conditions

From the chromosomal nature of sex determination, it is obvious that diseases due to recessive genes on the X chromosome will occur differentially in the two sexes. If a woman carries a recessive gene on one of her X chromosomes, its effect is likely to be masked by the normal allele of her other X chromosome. If, however, a male carries a recessive gene on his X chromosome, it cannot be masked and he will show the disorder. Hence the pedigrees of sex-linked recessive disorders are quite characteristic, with the disease appearing in males, and seeming to skip the carrier females of the intervening generations. Amongst such conditions which occur in males and practically never in females are the severe Duchenne muscular dystrophy, haemophilia (factor 8 deficiency), red/green colour blindness, Fabry's disease, Lever's optic atrophy, and many others.

However, there are several conditions due to a gene on an autosome which are expressed more in one sex than in another, and such conditions are said to be sex limited. In primary haemochromatosis there is increased absorption of iron from the intestine with subsequent deposition in the liver, pancreas, adrenals and other organs, and this condition is almost always limited to males, since in women menstruation counterbalances the increased iron absorption, and where women are affected there is always a history of oligomenorrhoea. Familial periodic paralysis, a disorder in the contractivity of muscle resulting from excess aldosterone, occurs in males more often than in females. In the opposite direction, fewer males than females are affected in Alport's syndrome (hereditary nephropathy with deafness). But in some cases it is difficult to distinguish whether the gene responsible is located on an autosome or a chromosome. In pseudohypoparathyroidism females are affected twice as often as males, which suggests that this disorder is due to an X-linked dominant, but against this it can be argued that hemizygous males are not more severely affected than heterozygous females, and a recent report suggests male to male transmission, which would be impossible if the gene is on the X chromosome. In testicular feminization, thanks to the presence of a single gene, persons who are chromosomally male develop into females, externally indistinguishable from normal females.

Chromosomal

Disorders chromosomal in origin (i.e. the sex chromosomes) affect the two sexes differentially. Turner's syndrome of course only occurs in those who are externally female, Kleinefelter's in those externally male, both intersexes. Ovarian dysgenesis cases (not Turner's) are often mosaics, usually of cell lines 45 XO/46 XX, again limited to external females, while the deviant behaviour that is associated in some cases of 47 XYY karyotype is of course restricted to external males.

Complex

However, it is in the disorders of multifactorial etiology, in which the genetic component is important but complex, that one finds many puzzling sex differences in susceptibility. Here the manifestation of the predisposing genotype depends upon sex modification. For example, in pyloric stenosis, Carter (1961) reported that between 1920 and 1940 there were treated at the Hospital for Sick Children, London, 774 males and 145 females, in all of whom the diagnosis had been confirmed by Ramstedt's operation. In our Newcastle series of over 500 facial cleft patients, cleft palate alone shows a preponderance in females, almost twice as many as in males, while cleft lip with or without cleft palate shows a predominance in males, thereby demonstrating the distinctness of the two conditions (Table II). Congenital heart disorders also show quite pronounced sex differences (Table III); coarctation of the aorta and tetralogy of Fallot both tend to have a strong male preponderance. Talipes equinovarus tends to occur twice as frequently in males as in females, ankylosing spondylitis six times as frequently; congenital dislocation of the hip and anencephaly tend to occur more often in females than in males. Such variation in sex ratio is particularly useful in the genetic analysis of such disorders, for they provide one of the more useful tests of the polygenic hypothesis of inheritance.

UNEQUAL ENVIRONMENTAL FACTORS

The hazards of occupation provide many clear examples of male preponderance of disease. The colic of lead poisoning was first described by Hippocrates in 370 B.C., poisoning by mercury, arsenic, manganese, nickel, chromium and other metals were an accompaniment to indus-

TABLE II

Newcastle upon Tyne facial cleft series number of cases by sex

	Male		Female		Sex ratio	
Cleft palate	50		97		52	
Cleft lip	67		49		137	
Cleft lip with cleft palate	131	198	77	126	170	157

TABLE III

Newcastle upon Tyne congenital heart series by sex

	Male	Female	Sex ratio
Coarctation of th aorta	65	35	186
Tetralogy of Fallot	60	40	150

trial development in this country and elsewhere, notably occurring in men who were involved in their extraction or utilization in industrial processes. Poisoning by organic compounds affected workers in a wide variety of industries from the preparation of synthetic dyes and perfumes to soap and detergent-making, and here there was differential spread outside the factories to those involved in application of insecticides. Particularly male again are the dust diseases of the lungs, silicosis the most important, not only in the quarrying, mining and dressing industries, but also in foundries and potteries. Occupational diseases of the skin involve women more than men in specific cases; the continuing use of soap and synthetic detergents, the use of cleansing solutions, polishes and preservatives makes the housewife, nurses and hairdressers particularly liable to sensitization dermatitis; the same occurs in girls who peel and squeeze oranges and lemons, and in those who sort/pack tulip bulbs, and, in the old days, in milkmaids who became sensitized by the poison from the cowslip family carried on the udders of the cow.

In most such conditions, with increased knowledge of industrial medicine and preventive action, the prevalence of the disease drops and so does the sex morbidity difference. But despite modern knowledge too many still remain. For instance, antibodies to Micropolyspora faeni which causes farmer's lung were found in 35 out of 124 males tested, but in only six out of 59 females (Morgan *et al.*, 1973), in an agricultural community in the south-west. Men dying in 1952–66 who had worked in the newspaper printing industry showed a pronounced excess of deaths from cancer of the lung and bronchus (Moss *et al.*, 1972). Insulation workers (i.e. exposed to asbestos) in Belfast showed X-ray abnormalities in 13 per cent of men who had worked for less than 10 years, increasing to 85 per cent in men who had spent more than 30 years in the industry (Langlands *et al.*, 1971). But there is a second factor in operation causing the sex differential to diminish—the changed pattern of occupation of the sexes today, and the arrival of women in the factories. For example, female asbestos workers showed a similarly increased respiratory morbidity and mortality in relation to length and severity of exposure (Newhouse *et al.*, 1972) as occurs in males. Once again the precise sex profile of morbidity depends upon the environment, particularly the social, in which people live.

The curious interplay of environmental factors in producing morbidity differentials is well shown by atherosclerosis, fatty degeneration of the artery walls, which is much more common in men than in women. The probability that an individual will develop this is correlated with the level of β-lipoprotein in his blood; males in the third decade of life show a rapid rise in cholesterol levels whereas females show a more gentle increase until the late 40s. This morbidity difference is partly self-inflicted. Cigarette smoking for the first few decades of this century was primarily a male prerogative and smoking induces acceleration of atherosclerosis. In recent decades women have tended to catch up in smoking habits, so we can expect a reduction in the sex differential on this account. Fashions in physique, attained by dietary habits and particularly differential consumption of saturated fats of animal origin which affect cholesterol levels, are also partly responsible. The slim figure fashion for women that started in the early 1920s led to a decline in obesity in women and not in men. For example, in the United States between 1900 and 1940, for females aged 25–35 the average weight for a given height decreased by 2–3 pounds, whereas for males there was an increase. The lack of exercise is another relevant environmental variable. But the sex difference in western society is not entirely due to such curious habits. For in women oestrogens apparently exert a protective effect, effective until the menopause, which accounts for the quite large sex differences in the serum cholesterol levels in mid-adulthood, and this difference is quite unrelated to the environmental differences.

EQUAL ENVIRONMENTS

It is not easy to distinguish conditions with sex-specific prevalences in which the environmental factors can be regarded as equal in the two sexes, and in many such conditions there is some genetic element to which a sex difference is often the first clue, so there is overlap with our first category. At the simplest level, in tasks involving finger mobility in later life (e.g. buttoning and unbuttoning, tying shoe laces), more females than males have difficulty, and this is particularly so in those over the age of 50 rather than below (Acheson *et al.*, 1973). This is the tip of the iceberg of the various forms of arthritis which show sex differences. Benign polyarthritis, arising commonly in young people between the ages of 5–24, and Still's disease occur more often in females than males. The chronic form of rheumatoid arthritis is similarly much more frequent in females than in males, some 2·5 times as great (Lawrence, 1969). The greater fragility of bone in the female elderly, reflecting the sex difference in patterns of bone growth and absorption, is well shown by the many studies of the incidence of fractures of the femoral neck, the upper humerus, and Potts' and Colles' fractures, all of which show an incidence above the age of 55 some two or three times as high in females as that in males (Eddy, 1972). Many such diseases show an age-specific prevalence. One finds a tendency for the prevalence curve of one sex to lag behind that of the other. For instance, with Dupuytren's contracture the female curve of age-specific prevalence lags about 10 years behind that of the male (Early, 1962). For osteoarthrosis of the proximal interphalangeal joints, the male curve lags some five years behind that of the female (Lawrence *et al.*, 1966). But again the mechanism by which the sex difference in the inexorable progress in prevalence with advancing years is brought about is far from clear.

Among the diseases that fall into this category, where no environmental influence can be held responsible, the cancers show remarkable sex differences. Men always have a higher incidence of cancer than women, other than cancers of the reproductive organs and a few other exceptions (Shimkin, 1965; Ashley, 1969a). For primary liver cancer in Singapore the ratio men:women is 7:1 (Toh, 1973), in Liverpool 5:1 (Doll *et al.*, 1956). Men develop lung cancer more frequently than women (the sex ratio male:female ranging from 1·5:1 to 9:1), and though this is partly due to the sex difference in cigarette smoking, and the different external social environments, it also occurs in men who are non-smokers (Haenszel and Taeuber, 1964). Among surgically treated patients with localized cancer of the lung, the survival rate is substantially higher in women than in men (Connelly *et al.*, 1966). Commoner in men than in women are cancers of the lip, buccal cavity, pharynx and oesophagus (Millar, 1961); of the skin, except melanoma (Carmichael, 1961; Carmichael and Silverstone, 1961); of the rectum (Ederer *et al.*, 1961; Ashley, 1970); of the pancreas (Muir, 1961); and of the bladder (Ashley, 1969b). In contrast to these male predominances, women tend to be more susceptible to cancer of the large intestine and of the thyroid (Meyer, 1962; Stocks, 1969).

As mentioned, the sex difference in the incidence of cancer may be partly due to the different environments in which the two sexes live and work, and particularly to increased male exposure to industrial carcinogenic substances. But that this is not the total explanation is shown by an excursion outside our own culture, with particular reference to hepatic cancers. A higher incidence of liver cancer in males is found in non-industrialized countries; moreover, the incidence is lower in Europe and North America than in Africa and Asia. Alcoholism frequently produces liver damage, and social factors that result in higher consumption of alcohol by men that women make for male predominance in the incidence of liver cancer. This is certainly not the case in the Far East, where Malay men and women consume the same foods, men take very little alcohol, and yet men still have a greater incidence of liver cancer than women. Thirdly, animal work indicates a male preponderance of hepatic tumour in mice—who neither smoke nor drink. Animal experiments suggest that sex organs are involved in the sex difference in hepatocarcinogenesis. Either the presence of testosterone induces hepatic tumours, or the presence of oestrogen protects the liver against tumour development, and the evidence appears to favour the former. The thyroid is also involved, and possibly other endocrine glands, mediating the effect of testosterone (Toh, 1973). It appears that while environmental factors are to some extent responsible for the higher incidence of cancer in males than in females, they are far from being totally responsible and though the cause of most cancers is still not understood, in their metabolic activation the sex difference in hormonal pattern may well be a primary importance and hence responsible for the curious sex distribution.

A conspicuous group of disorders differentially represented between the sexes is that of the psychiatric illnesses. For the British population, those expected to have some psychiatric disorder at some time during their life are estimated as 11 per cent for the male population and 17 per cent for the female, though interpretation of these figures is not straightforward on account of the sex difference in prison committals by the courts for crimes by psychopaths. In the United States in 1966–68 women comprised at least 60 per cent of the adult population in psychiatric facilities, and most recent studies indicate that two-thirds of psychiatric patients, either in hospital or outpatients, are women. For schizophrenia Slater's (1971) figures on first admissions to mental hospitals per million of population, England and Wales 1952–60, showed that males were in excess of females at ages 15–35, but thereafter the female admission rates were strongly in excess. In the affective psychoses (1966) and in the depressive psychoses (1964–66), admission rates for females are consistently and conspicuously heavier than for males at all age groups. The expectation of manic depressive illness in the general population across north-west Europe shows the conspicuous female excess in every country.

Such differences probably indicate the presence of the genetic element that underlies these. Yet it is all too easy to overlook the effect of the complexity of the life of a woman today, the need for continuing adaptation to the changes that occur in its normal course; many indeed adapt successfully, others only at some cost. At the adolescent stage there may occur in a girl the awareness of the need for choice between profession and domesticity; in some adolescent girls little difficulty arises, others assume a non-competitive role in relation to boys, while others at this stage become depressed, withdrawn, attempt suicide, or work out their frustrations in some other way. With the arrival of pregnancy and motherhood comes the necessity for the women to interrupt a career and change her role; stress will develop, particularly if this decision is made unwillingly, and if she feels the loss of her personal independence. The anxiety and physical changes that occur in pregnancy are superimposed. The physiological changes accompanying childbirth and heightened emotional difficulties may lead to severe depressive episodes or post-partum psychoses. During the problem years of child-rearing, many women experience a sense of failure, a sense of isolation, and the help they need is concealed in terms of complaints and backache, tiredness, sleeplessness, and others. When the children become more independent and leave home, the role for which the woman may have sacrificed her career is no longer required, and again there is the feeling of emptiness. But it is with the fundamental body changes that occur at the menopause that the climax is reached, a time of discomfort, anxiety and stress, when the whole biological rhythm is being readjusted, a time when all too many are advised "to let nature take its course" or tranquillizers provide a convenient way of shelving individual physical and emotional difficulties. It is not surprising that the admission rates for the psychoses in females reach their peak in the menopausal age group. But since the female excess occurs at all ages, and the final step to the peak is relatively slight, this is clearly not the sole explanation. Moreover it seems unlikely that the stresses are more than triggers for some deeper disturbance of a more delicately balanced equilibrium, which with the stresses of modern life is upset more easily.

CONDITIONS RELATING TO THE SEX ORGANS

Here first are the developmental disorders and infections of childhood. Hypospadias, undescended testicles, balanitis, are peculiar to the male, and inguinal hernia is much commoner in the male than in the female. On the other hand, vulvovaginitis is peculiar to the female, while urinary infections of childhood are considerably commoner in girls.

In adulthood there occurs the whole range of gynaecological disorders which are obviously sex-specific, but serving special mention is the curious distribution of the malignant tumours of the sex organs. There is a far higher incidence of ovarian and uterine cancers than there are of testis and prostate cancers. Why are they so common, and why do they show the strange reversal in sex incidence by comparison with almost every other cancer? While the difference is not surprising in view of the great difference in anatomical structure and physiological function, it is still not understood; perhaps it may be attributed to the recurrent cyclic stimulation of these organs in females rather than in males.

One last topic that deserves mention under this heading is the trend that is occurring in venereal diseases. In Britain the ratio of male:female cases of gonorrhoea in 1965 was 3·2:1 (Ministry of Health, 1966). In 1973 the ratio of male:female cases was reduced to 1·8:1. The number of cases in women has risen by 61 per cent in five years, particularly in the 18–19-year-old age group (Department of Health and Social Security, 1974). This is obviously due to the change in standards, particularly in young people, for today far too many of these cases occur in "affluent, good-time, easy amateurs" rather than the old professional prostitutes (Wigfield, 1972). But the change is particularly tragic, on account of the serious risk to impairment of consequent fertility where the gonococcal infection extends to the fallopian tubes, and this infertility is likely to be distressing in subsequent adult life. Many of the young girls are unaware of the risks (Department of Health and Social Security 1972), believing that venereal disease is curable, and fear has been replaced by indifference. It is not appreciated that the scars of the cured infection remain, and it is these that are the basis of subsequent infertility.

Mortality Differences

It is often thought that male fetuses are more susceptible to antenatal death than females. Relatively few studies have been made, but the facts so far do not seem to support this. Table IV shows these ratios of spontaneous abortuses in relation to karyotype and trimester of abortion. Those of normal karyotype show up no significant excess of either male or female deaths in the total series, or in the first or second trimester. These data relate only to series in which full karyotyping was carried

TABLE IV

Sex of spontaneous abortuses

Trimester	Normal karyotype XY	XX	Sex Ratio
1st	24	28	86
2nd	16	11	146
Unstated	131	155	85
TOTAL	171	194	88

From Geneva Conference 1966.

out, and not those in which the sex was identified by the less reliable sex chromatin examination alone. If spontaneous abortuses of abnormal karyotype are also included, the sex ratio again remains very close to unity. Perhaps the difference from the earlier view is due to the early reliance on morphological sexing of abortuses, notoriously difficult.

When we come to perinatal mortality we are on surer ground, thanks to the magnificent perinatal mortality survey (Butler and Bonham, 1963; Butler and Alberman, 1969). In this, every birth in the country during the week 3–9 March 1958 was monitored to give population information, and then data on stillbirths and neonatal deaths continued to be collected throughout the months of March, April and May of that year. The national survey covered some 17,000 births and the death statistics some 7,600. This study showed conclusively a higher male perinatal mortality. Male infants made up 51·7 per cent of the population and accounted for 55·3 per cent of the deaths. Examining the data by gestational age (Table V), higher male mortality is seen for all except

TABLE V

Perinatal mortality survey
Sex ratio of deaths by gestation groups

Gestation	Sex ratio (male:female) in all births	Sex ratio (male:female) in deaths
Under 28 weeks	1·00	1·35
28–31	0·80	1·27
32–35	1·27	1·23
36–37	1·18	1·28
38–39	1·12	1·23
40–41	1·05	1·32
42+	1·00	1·13
ALL	1·07	1·25

TABLE VI

Perinatal mortality survey
Sex ratio of deaths by birthweight groups

Birthweight (gm)	Sex ratio (male: female) in all births	Sex ratio (male: female) in deaths
< 1,000	0·78	1·10
1,001–1,500	0·90	0·98
1·501–2·000	1·01	1·15
2,001–2,500	0·81	1·33
2,501–3,000	0·74	1·20
3,001–3,500	0·92	1·29
3,501–4,000	1·40	1·69
4001 +	1·76	2·15
ALL	1·07	1·25

one gestation group; the excess of male deaths occurs primarily in those of higher birth weights (Table VI). This male excess mortality is consistent across almost the whole range of findings of primary necropsy (Table VII), though it is less marked in deaths from isoimmunization

TABLE VII

Perinatal mortality survey
Sex ratio by primary necropsy findings

Primary necropsy finding	Male	Female
Congenital malformations	0·6	1·0
Isoimmunization	1·2	1·0
Early neonatal death (no histological lesion)	1·2	1·0
Antepartum death (no major lesion) and antepartum anoxia	1·3	1·0
Intrapartum anoxia	1·3	1·0
Intrapartum anoxia with cerebral birth trauma	1·8	1·0
Cerebral birth trauma	1·8	1·0
Hyaline membrane	1·8	1·0
Intraventricular haemorrhage	1·8	1·0
Massive pulmonary haemorrhage	2·1	1·0
Pulmonary infection	2·5	1·0
Total population born (16,994)	1·1	1·0
March perinatal deaths (617)	1·3	1·0

and also for early neonatal death without histological lesion. It is probably justifiable to attribute at least a small proportion of the excess of male deaths due to birth injury, asphyxia and atelectasis to the fact that the male infant at birth is on average slightly larger and has a slightly greater head circumference than the female, and there is greater mechanical difficulty. The only female excess occurs in deaths with congenital malformations. But even in these the sex distribution depends on the type of lesion. Among cases of anencephalus, 340 were female, 149 male. Deaths from malformations of the gastrointestinal tract were particularly pronounced in boys (75 boys to 36 girls); similarly, deaths from malformations of the renal system occurred in 115 boys, 45 girls (Table VIII). These sex differences are in keeping with almost all other reports.

TABLE VIII

Perinatal mortality survey
Malformations of the renal system
*March, April and May 1958 deaths (7,117 singletons)**

Malformation of Kidney	Number of cases	Male	Female	Sex Male to female ratio
Bilateral agenesis	23†	16	5	3·2
Unilateral agenesis	17‡	10	6	1·7
Hypoplasia	19	13	6	2·2
Large cystic	28	21	7	3·0
Small cystic	18	13	5	2·6
Horseshoe	14	9	5	1·8
Hydronephrosis	44	33	11	3·0
Control week population	16,994			1·1

* Excluding mongols, anencephalics and cases of spina bifida.
† Sex not known in two.
‡ Sex not known in one.

Sex mortality differentials persist throughout life. In childhood, road accidents furnish a striking example. In these, after the age of one year the male preponderance in mortality is very great, due to the increased incidence of accidents in boys. This discrepancy may be attributed to the timidity or caution of the girl or to the carelessness or adventure of the boy. In adulthood come the hazards of occupation, where morbidity has already been discussed, which provide many clear examples of male preponderance of disease-specific mortality.

But there is one sex-specific occupational hazard which was very real in earlier days. If one traces back an ascendant pedigree in a rural area of a present-day young adult for three generations so that it includes two parents, four grandparents, and eight great-grandparents, about

1 in 10 of such pedigrees show at least one death in childbirth or some associated disorder in the first month thereafter. This is not a true incidence figure for it relates only to those families in which offspring survive, and of course the death may have occurred at the birth of a sib later than the individual in the pedigree. When we enumerate our present-day worries, we all too frequently overlook the blessings that today has brought, and for women surely one of the greatest must be the freedom from fear of death in childbirth.

However, it is the changing pattern of sex differences in mortality that is of particular interest. There has been a spectacular fall in mortality in western countries in the last 200 years, during which expectation of life at birth has more than doubled from about 35 to nearly 75 years. This spectacular mortality decline has not been equally shared by the two sexes. No matter to which country we look, the pattern emerges. Table IX shows the age standardized death rates for the United States, England and Wales, and New Zealand, this century.

TABLE IX
Standardized death rate

		M	F	Δ(M−F)
United States	1910	24·30	21·18	3·12
	1930	19·74	16·74	3·00
	1950	15·24	10·74	4·51
	1965	14·49	8·95	5·54
England and Wales	1911	23·77	19·54	4·23
	1930	18·95	14·90	4·04
	1950	15·61	11·02	4·59
	1965	14·63	8·85	5·78
New Zealand	1911	17·69	14·75	2·94
	1930	15·75	13·22	2·53
	1950	14·01	10·64	3·37
	1965	13·97	8·98	4·98

All three show

a consistently elevated male mortality,
a steady decline in both sexes,
and increasing difference between males and females.

The same trend can be shown in a different way by the expectation of life at birth (Table X). The first and second have long been known. For example, Stolnitz's (1956) review showed that sex mortality differentials favoured females in most countries at all ages except primarily the

TABLE X

Expectation of life at birth

		M	F	Δ(F−M)
United States	1910	48·46	52·01	3·55
	1930	57·31	60·70	3·39
	1950	65·30	70·92	5·62
	1965	66·88	73·87	6·99
England and Wales	1911	49·35	53·38	4·03
	1930	59·02	63·27	4·25
	1950	66·57	71·32	4·75
	1965	68·53	74·79	6·26
New Zealand	1911	60·27	63·12	2·85
	1930	64·36	67·26	2·90
	1950	68·39	72·22	3·83
	1965	68·78	74·65	5·87

reproductive ages; exceptions included the 7–17 age group in some nineteenth century European populations, and other ages in some Latin-America, African and Asian countries up till the 1950s. El Badry (1969) noted that in India, Pakistan and Ceylon, male life expectancy at birth exceeded that of females until at least the early 1960s.

Let us look first at the ages at which the sex differential is most marked. Figure 1 shows that between 1910 and 1965 in the United States, the male/female difference in age-specific mortality declined

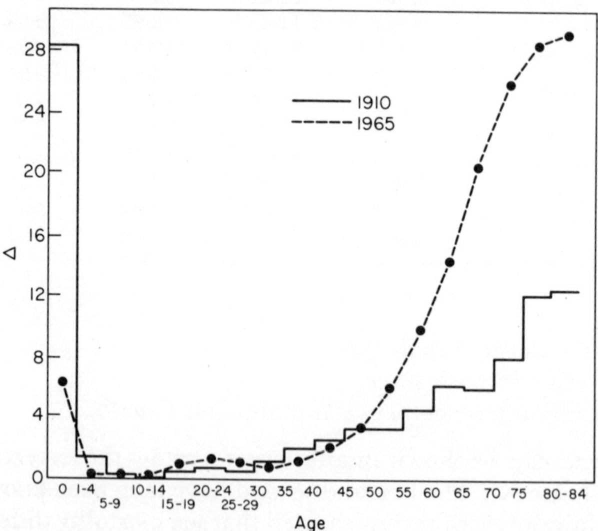

FIG. 1. Sex difference in age-specific mortality rates (M-F) USA (rate per thousand).

sharply below the age of 5, from 28 per thousand to 6 per thousand. There was relatively little change between the ages of 5 and 49, but from the age of 50 onwards there was a sharp increase. The changes in the under-five age group decreased the sex difference, and these were brought about by the improved control of infectious and parasitic diseases, the improved knowledge and treatment of children with congenital disorders, failure to thrive, low birth weight, and general debility. The relatively slight change in the ages 5–49, the age group in which maternal mortality related to child-bearing occurred, indicates either that the contribution of maternal mortality in 1910 must have been small or, more likely, that a substantial decline in maternal mortality with better care of women in labour, was accompanied by a similar decline in male mortality, for example from industrial accidents. It is the changes above the age of 50 that account for virtually all of the overall increase in excess male mortality and, for these, prime responsibility must certainly be cardiovascular and renal diseases and cancer. In the United States in 1960, cardiovascular and renal diseases accounted for 66·1 per cent, malignant neoplasms for 15·3 per cent of total deaths above age 50.

A recent study by Retherford (1975) has attempted to partition the change in the sex mortality difference 1910–65 in the United States. Looking first at the different age groups (Table XI), in 1910 the major

TABLE XI

Contributions to the sex difference in standardized mortality and its change 1910–1965

	United States			England and Wales			New Zealand		
Age	1910	1965	1910–65	1910	1965	1910–65	1910	1965	1910–65
0–19	20·2	3·6	−17·8	14·1	2·8	—28·1	10·2	3·5	−6·2
20–39	8·1	4·9	0·7	5·5	2·1	−7·2	−0·1	4·4	10·8
40–59	28·2	24·9	20·8	22·3	17·1	2·7	21·3	18·2	13·9
60–79	36·3	57·6	85·2	45·7	62·9	109·8	47·2	59·9	78·2
80+	7·3	9·0	11·1	12·3	15·1	22·8	21·4	14·0	3·4
TOTAL	100·0	100·0	100·0	100·0	100·0	100·0	100·0	100·0	100·0
	(3·12)	(5·54)	(2·42)	(4·23)	(5·78)	(1·55)	(2·94)	(4·98)	(2·05)

contributions to the sex difference in mortality were in the 60–79, the 40–59 and the 0–19 groups. In 1965 the 60–79 group had established a far greater lead over the other ages, the 40–59 still accounted for about 25 per cent of the difference, but this time the childhood differences made the least contribution. Turning to the increase in sex difference from 1910–65 (Table XII), this is almost entirely due to the 60–79 year

TABLE XII

Contributions to the sex difference in standardized mortality and its change 1910–1965

Cause	United States			England and Wales			New Zealand		
	1910	1965	1910–65	1910	1965	1910–65	1910	1965	1910–65
Infection	18·2	1·5	–20·1	13·9	1·2	–33·3	2·5	1·1	–0·9
Cardiovascular-renal	41·1	55·0	73·0	19·2	47·1	123·2	24·7	53·0	93·5
Neoplasms	–21·1	12·7	56·3	–3·2	19·7	82·1	–3·7	13·6	38·5
Respiratory	4·1	9·3	16·1	20·7	22·2	26·2	16·6	15·9	14·7
Digestion	6·0	4·2	1·8	6·2	2·2	–8·7	1·9	2·4	3.2
Maternal	–7·8	–0·2	9·6	–3·6	–0·2	9·2	–6·4	– 0·2	8·8
Early infancy	4·9	1·3	–3·5	3·2	0·9	–5·3	3·3	0·9	–2·7
Accident	42·2	12·7	–25·5	15·2	4·8	–23·6	34·2	9·3	–26·4
Other	12·4	3·6	–7·7	28·4	2·1	–69·8	26·8	4·1	–28·6
TOTAL	100·0	100·0	100·0	100·0	100·0	100·0	100·0	100·0	100·0
	(3·12)	(5·54)	(2·42)	(4·23)	(5·78)	(1·55)	(2·94)	(4·98)	(2·05)

age group, while the childhood mortality has tended to reduce the sex difference. Examining now the particular causes, in 1910 the greater part of the sex mortality difference was due to accidents and cardiovascular and renal diseases; neoplasms tended to reduce the excess male mortality, and so did maternal deaths. By 1965 while cardiovascular and renal disorders accounted for the greater part of the sex mortality differential, the effect of neoplasms was reversed, that of accidents had dropped appreciably, and that of maternal deaths had practically disappeared. The greatest part of the change in the sex mortality difference over the period is accounted for by the cardiovascular and renal disorders, followed by the neoplasms, but accidents and infections have tended to reduce the difference. The same pattern is shown in the other two countries examined. Figure 2 shows diagrammatically the results

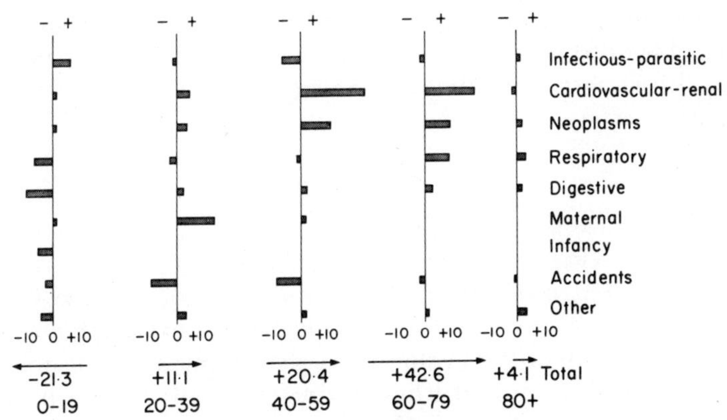

FIG. 2. Contribution of causes of death, by age, to the change in sex difference in expectation of life $\Delta(e^f_0 - e_0m)$ 1910–1965.

relating to expectation of life at birth. The units are arbitrary, but internally comparable. They show the same importance of cardiovascular and renal disorders and the neoplasms in accounting for the secular change in sex differential. These findings are in agreement with others in the literature. Ciocco (1940) showed the importance of circulatory and respiratory disorders for the sex mortality difference in US whites; Moriyama and Woolsey (1951) showed how changes in cardiovascular and renal diseases were increasing the female mortality advantage, and Dorn (1961) the chronic respiratory disorders. Enterline (1961) showed that the increased male mortality between 1920 and 1960 was due to different causes in different age groups. Decline in female death rates for tuberculosis, maternal mortality and increase in males from motor vehicle accidents were primarily responsible for the changes in 15–24 age group. Decline in female deaths from cancer of the uterus and increase in male deaths from cancer of the lung, coronary heart disease, and diseases associated with high blood pressure, were important causes for the 45–64 age group.

This change in the sex difference in mortality has produced a series of consequences of social importance. First there is the numerical disparity of men and women at older ages and its effect on marital chances. Although more males are born than females, differential death rates turn this surplus into a deficit in the later ages, a deficit that is increasing. In a monogamous society, a high proportion of older women remain unmarried. By 1970 in the United States, at ages 50–59 there were two unmarried women to every unmarried man, and at ages 60–69 there were nearly three. Other social effects of this trend are the increasing incidence of widowhood and the economic cost of excess male mortality and ill health at ages of maximum earning power. The cost of these has to be met by society.

Conclusion

It is clearly impossible to review comprehensively the numerous sex inequalities in disease and their resulting effect on mortality. What has been attempted here is to show that wide ranging though these are, they are essentially part of the spectrum of biological differences between the sexes, consequent upon the evolutionary development of the sex polymorphism to the degree that it has attained in man; that in part they derive from the innate biological differences between the sexes that develop as a result of the genetic instructions with which the individual is endowed at conception; but that in part they stem from circumstances of modern man's own making. Whatever their origin, however, the trend to increasing sex differential in mortality will bring increasing demands on the social services involved with the elderly.

References

Acheson, R. M. and Ginsburg, G. N. (1973). New Haven survey of joint diseases. XVI. Impairment, disability and arthritis. *Br. J. prev. soc. Med.* **27**, 168–176.

Ashley, D. J. B. (1969a). A male-female differential in tumour incidence. *Br. J. Cancer* **23**, 21–25.

Ashley, D. J. B. (1969b). Sex differences in the incidence of tumours at various sites. *Br. J. Cancer* **23**, 26–30.

Ashley, D. J. B. (1970). A systematic sex difference in intestinal carcinoma. *Cancer* **25**, 966–971.

Butler, N. R. and Alberman, E. (1969). *Perinatal Problems*. Edinburgh: Livingstone.

Butler, N. R. and Bonham, D. G. (1963). *Perinatal Mortality*. Edinburgh: Livingstone.

Carmichael, G. G. (1961). The epidemiology of skin cancers in Queensland: the significance of premalignant conceptions. *Br. J. Cancer* **15**, 425–428.

Carmichael, G. G. and Silverstone, H. (1961). The epidemiology of skin cancer, in Queensland: the incidence. *Br. J. Cancer* **15**, 409–424.

Carter, C. O. (1961). The inheritance of congenital pyloric stenosis. *Br. Med. Bull.* **17**, 251–253.

Challis, J. R. G., Robinson, J. S., Rurak, D. W. and Thorburn, G. D. (1975). The development of endocrine function in the human fetus. In *Biology of Human Fetal Growth*. Edited by D. F. Roberts and A. M. Thomson. London: Taylor and Francis.

Ciocco, A. (1940). Sex differentials in morbidity and mortality. *Q. Rev. Biol.* **15**, 59–73, 192–210.

Connelly, R. R., Cutler, S. J. and Baylis, P. (1966). *J. nat. Cancer Inst.* **36**, 277–287.

Department of Health and Social Security (1972). *On the State of the Public Health, Annual Report of the Chief Medical Officer for the Year* **1971**, p. 69. London: Her Majesty's Stationery Office.

Department of Health and Social Security (1974). *On the State of the Public Health, Annual Report of the Chief Medical Officer for the Year* **1973**, p. 48. London: Her Majesty's Stationery Office.

Doll, R., Payne, P. and Waterhouse, J. (1956). *Cancer Incidence in Five Continents*. Berlin and New York: Springer-Verlag.

Dorn, H. F. (1961). The increasing mortality from chronic respiratory diseases. In *Proceedings of the Social Statistics Section of the American Statistical Association*, 148–152.

Early, P. F. (1962). Population studies in Dupuytren's contracture. *J. Bone Jt. Surg.* **44B**, 602–613.

Eddy, T. P. (1972). Deaths from domestic falls and fractures. *Br. J. prev. soc. Med.* **26**, 173–179.

Ederer, R., Cutler, S. J., Eisenberg, H. and Keogh, J. R. (1961). Survival of patients with cancer of the large intestine and rectum. *J. nat. Cancer Inst.* **26**, 489–510.

El Badry, M. A. (1969). Higher female than male mortality in some countries in South Asia: a digest. *J. Amer. stat. Assoc.* **64**, 1234–1244.

Enterline, P. E. (1961). Causes of death responsible for recent increases in sex mortality differentials in the United States. *Milbank Memorial Fund Quarterly* **39**, 312–328.

Haenszel, W. and Taeuber, K. E. (1964). Lung cancer mortality as related to residence and smoking histories. II: white females. *J. nat. Cancer Inst.* **32**, 803–838.

Langlands, J. H. M., Wallace, W. F. and Simpson, M. J. C. (1971). Insulation workers in Belfast. 2: Morbidity in men still at work. *Br. J. industr. Med.* **28**, 217–225.

Lawrence, J. S. (1969). Epidemiology and genetics of rheumatoid arthritis. *Rhrumatology* **2**, 1.

Lawrence, J. S., Bremmer, J. M. and Bier, F. (1966). Osteo-arthrosis. *Prevalence in Ann. Rheum. Dis.* **25**, 1–24.

Marshall, W. A. (1970). Sex differences at puberty. *J. biosoc. Sci. Suppl* **2**, 31–41.

Meyer, P. C. (1962). The relationship between the nodular goitre and carcinoma of the thyroid. *Br. J. Cancer* **16**, 16–26.

Millar, I. B. (1961). Gastro-intestinal cancer and geochemistry in North Montgomeryshire. *Br. J. Cancer* **15**, 175–199.

Ministry of Health (1966). *On the State of Public Health, Annual Report of the Chief Medical Officer for the Year* **1965**, p. 80. London: Her Majesty's Stationery Office.

Morgan, D. C., Smyth, J. T., Lister, R. W. and Petlybridge, R. J. (1973). Chest symptoms and farmer's lung: a community survey. *Br. J. industr. Med.* **30**, 259–265.

Moriyama, I. M. and Woolsey, T. D. (1951). Statistical studies of heart disease. IX: Race and sex differences in cardiovascular-renal mortality from the major cardiovascular-renal diseases. *Publ. Hlth Rep.* **66**, 355–368.

Moss, E., Scott, T. S. and Atherley, G. R. L. (1972). Mortality of newspaper workers from lung cancer and bronchitis, 1952–66. *Br. J. industr. Med.* **29**, 1–14.

Muir, C. S. (1961). Cancer of the liver, pancreas and peritoneum in Singapore. *Br. J. Cancer* **15**, 30–40.

Newhouse, M. L., Berry, G., Wagner, J. C. and Turok, M. E. (1972). A study of the mortality of female asbestos workers. *Br. J. industr. Med.* **29**, 134–141.

Retherford, R. D. (1975). *The Changing Sex Differential in Mortality*. Connecticut and London: Greenwood Press.

Reyes, F. I., Winter, J. S. D. and Faiman, C. (1973). Studies on human sexual developments. I: Fetal gonadal and adrenal sex steriods. *J. Clin. Endocr. Metab.* **37**, 74.

Reyes, F. I., Boroditsky, R. S., Winter, J. S. D. and Faiman, C. (1974). Studies on human sexual developments. II: Fetal and maternal serum gonadotropin and sex steroid concentrations. *J. Clin. Endocr. Metab.* **38**, 612.

Roberts, D. F., Triger, D. R. and Morgan, R. J. (1966). Glucose-6-phosphate dehydrogenase deficiency and haemoglobin level in Jamaican children. *West Indies Med. J.* **19**, 204–211.

Shimkin, M. B. (1965). Epidemiology of cancer: spatial-temporal aggregation. *Cancer Res.* **25**, 1363–1374.

Slater, E. and Cowie, V. (1971). *The Genetics of Mental Disorders*. London: Oxford University Press.

Stocks, P. (1969). Female susceptibility to cancer and other diseases indicated by British and European mortality rates. *Br. J. Cancer* **23**, 254–268.

Stolnitz, G. J. (1956). A century of international mortality trends: II. *Population Studies* **10**, 17–42.

Tanner, J. M. (1962). *Growth at Adolescence*. Second edition. Oxford: Blackwell.

Toh, Y. C. (1973). Physiological and biochemical reviews of sex differences and carcinogenesis with particular reference to the liver. In *Advances in Cancer Research*. Edited by G. Klein and S. Weinhouse. New York and London: Academic Press.

Wigfield, A. S. (1972). 27 years of uninterrupted contact tracing "The Tyneside Scheme". *Br. J. Ven. Dis.* **48**, 37.

Single Factor Predisposition to Disease

J. H. EDWARDS

The Infant Development Unit,
Queen Elizabeth Medical Centre, Birmingham, England

The basic understanding of single factor disposition to disease was one of the major triumphs of the first half of this century, bounded by the one factor one ferment prediction of Garrod and Bateson and the one gene one enzyme confirmation of Beadle and Tatum. There are still many unknowns. In the dominant disorders in man, in particular, we are still ignorant of the nature of the offending factor and the mechanism of its offence. However, notwithstanding numerous statements to the contrary, dominant disorders due to factors beyond optical microscopy are a less common form of human disability than recessives, and I will not consider them further. We may consider the nature of single-factor disposition to disease, and by single factor disposition I mean that the factor, or its absence, is sufficient for the development of the disease, in distinction to predisposition which implies a tendency only, with reference to a rough map (Fig. 1). This shows the nature of the action of the proteins, which act both as enzymes, the catalytic conveyors across molecular distances, and as moving conveyors, such as haemoglobins, which move substances physically either by diffusion or by active circulation.

Predisposition by some factor imposes a weaker relationship to disease, since of those predisposed only a proportion are afflicted, this proportion being determined by the combined effects of other factors, of the environment, and of chance. Geneticists who use numerical methods tend to equate chance with the environment: epidemiologists tend to equate it with the inborn constitution. However, the genetic material, both in development and in the later administration of the developed organism, is inadequate to do more than provide broad directives which will be buffeted by the vagaries of chance.

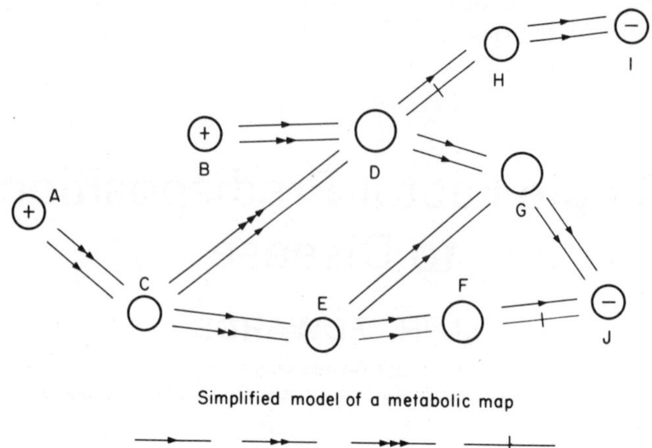

FIG. 1. Simple metabolic map showing metabolites A and B entering a series of synthetic pathways controlled by genetically determined enzymes —→—, —→→— —→→→ and —|— to give final products I and J.

As Dr Roberts has shown, sex provides a particularly simple example of single factor predisposition to disease. Sometimes, as in silicosis or carcinoma of the breast, no mathematical expertise is necessary to explain this difference, although even this field could be made difficult with a little ingenuity.

In such sex differences as the response of children to whooping-cough, which is more severe in girls, or the tendency to medulloblastoma, which is commoner in boys, the mechanism is clearly complex. The Y chromosome apparently protects or predisposes to everything to which the flesh is heir—but this is just another way of saying that boys and girls differ, and disease is but a breakdown of health.

An organism, or a part of an organism, such as a cell, can be regarded as a set of substances which are incremented and decremented by various intervening enzymatic activities. Basically these enzymes may be considered as consisting of two sets of molecules, which may be identical, and which are produced from the paternal and maternal genetic material.

The map (Fig. 1) shows this general form. Differences in amounts of different substances between different individuals in the same environment is due to different strengths of enzymes. It is these differences which lead to individuals being distinguishable, and even to species being distinguishable. If some substance is essential to normal living and is not produced, then abnormality arises. Similarly, if a failure to break down some substance leads to its reaching toxic levels, or to becoming a physical obstacle within the cell, abnormality again arises. This is the well-known chain effect which is shown in Fig. 2.

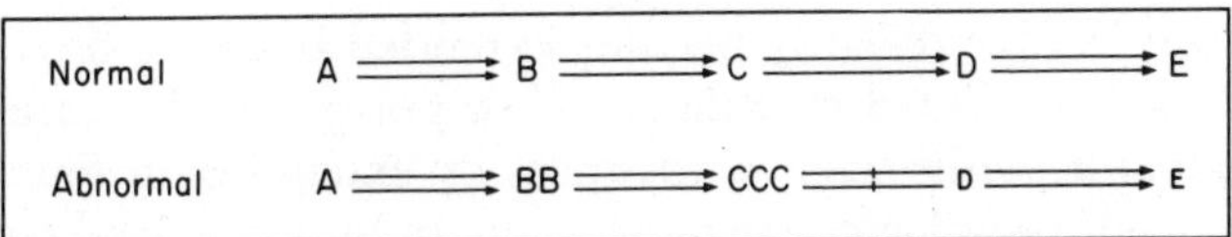

Fig. 2. Single-track enzymatic processes showing effect of "block". Each line represents the enzymes coded by genes from one parent.

If we look at the metabolic map in places where there are forks, leading to a net, it is easy to construct models in which a double defect is necessary for severe change in level. For example, if two loci A and B control enzymes relating to the formation or removal of some substance, the disease might occur only when both sets are defective, and we might have the consequence of various pairs (Fig. 3).

	BB	Bb	bb
AA	W	W	W
Aa	W	W	W
aa	W	W	I

Fig. 3. Showing possible results of a block when loci A and B provide enzymes which catalyse the same end product.

However,.both the alleles *a* and *b* would predispose to disease, in the sense that they would be common in the afflicted. This situation would be difficult to define by observation, since the sib incidence would be only 1 in 16. No clear examples are known in man.

Most disorders in man are less simple than the all-or-nothing effects of the enzymes on single track metabolic pathways; since all disorders are, in principle, capable of being defined in terms of the wrong levels of metabolites, and since all metabolites are determined by the basic restrictions of import, export and stock, it is difficult to see how any disorder can be unrelated to the genetic differences which distinguish us from one another in both health and disease.

Where the offending metabolite or group of metabolites is in the same region of the metabolic map, we may say that all neighbouring enzymes affect the metabolic level, and the neighbouring loci are the single loci which predispose to disease by a functional relationship to the offending metabolite.

These words have recently become extended by being used to define a set of disorders termed multifactorial or polygenic. This seems to me unfortunate, for, while science advances by extending its foundation of tautology, such tautologies are of no value in building on these foundations; to say a disorder is consequent on a single factor is meaningful: all disorders not dependant on a single factor are necessarily dependant on many factors, and to define the vast majority of disorders by an adjective which suggests to the unwary that it specifies a meaningful subset is likely to mislead, and has been responsible for such varied actions as the poor funding of studies of teratogens, especially in spina bifida, and, in the USA, to the diversion of funds needed for education to employing bus-drivers and psychologists.

All disorders are multifactorial or polygenic, although in some almost the whole of the variation is, for practical purposes, defined by a single locus.

The mechanism by which these loci produce their effect is, of course, as broad and variable as the whole canvas of disease—an even more variable and complex scenario than that provided by health. We may, however, document the more obvious situations in which a single locus may predispose to disease.

1. *Toxicity from high levels.* Tissues vary, and all have different optima for the levels of the nutritional medium they have to share. The joints suffer from high uric acid levels, the arteries from high cholesterol, the lens from high galactose, and, where a joint or a coronary artery is incommoded by such encrustations it is easy to overlook that such environments may be unusually good for other tissues. As might be expected, the levels of common metabolic substances, such as urea, cholesterol and glucose, are strongly related to disease susceptibility; the furring up of the arteries by cholesterol can even be incriminated in half the morbidity of man. Other forms of variation can lead to similar disease predisposition, such as pigmentation, are also due to many loci. Sunburn provides a simple example of a multifactorically determined, or polygenic, disorder, in this case of an optional nature. The response to cigarette smoking is probably similar. We all swallow several grammes of blood group substances in our daily gallon of saliva. It is hardly surprising that variation in these substances affects the risk of stomach disorders.

Of the many loci which affect such levels some are stronger than others. In principle it should be possible to define strong loci by the distribution of the levels in populations. In practice this is not so, since, by definition, the addition of normal curves tends to produce a normal curve, and antimodes are only produced under extreme condition (Figs 4 and 5). Even such an obvious predisposition of that of the Y chromosome to stature, and this adds almost six inches, or about 1·7 standard deviations, to the height, would be difficult to infer by studying populations whose individuals were unspecified by sex. The claim that strong loci are demonstrable as common determinants of cholesterol level must await the application of appropriate methods of analysis to adequate data.

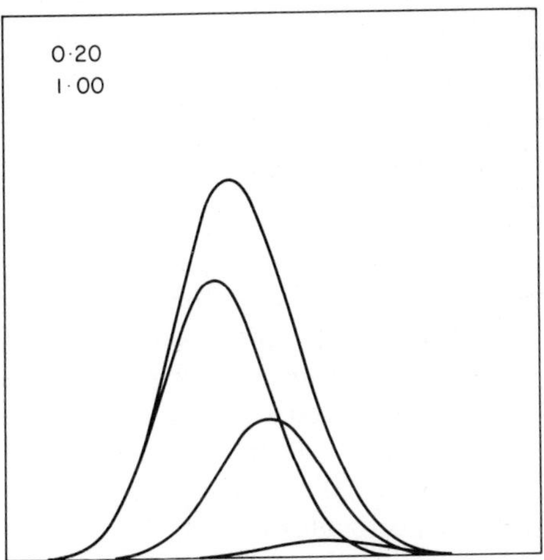

Fig. 4. Curve showing how three normal curves, the distribution of the three phenotypes due to alleles with proportion 0·2 and 0·8, and "effects" 1·0 standard deviation, combine to give a fairly normal distribution.

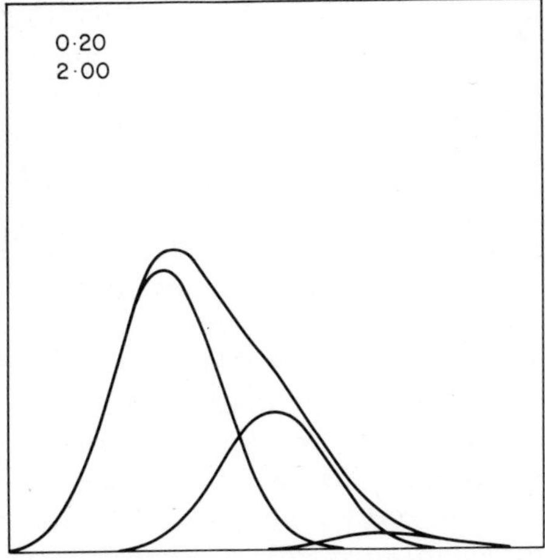

Fig. 5. As Fig. 4, but strength of allele increased to two units of standard deviation.

We may define the variation at any locus only under the artificial conditions of non-interaction with other loci, or the ideal of absence of other variation, an ideal which can be realised in the laboratory by inbreeding, but only at a cost of loss of relevance to what happens outside the laboratory.

We may define the influence of a locus with allele A with alleles 1, 2, . . . i etc. which have effects a_1, a_2, . . . a_i etc., and proportion p_1, p_2, . . . p_i etc. by such measures as

i. which locus has the strongest allele (at which locus are the most distinct homozygotes found),
ii. which locus has the most influential alleles (i.e. at which locus is the $\Sigma p_i d_i^2$ where d_i is the influence of an allele on the mean,
iii. which locus is necessary.

If we take the problem of sunburn we could, in principle, unravel the metabolic networks which define the synthesis of pigment, their response to light, and the independent mechanisms of repair. If, for simplicity, we merely consider the production-line for pigment we could say that, since at least two loci are necessary for pigment production, their absence leading to albinism, one leading to paler albinos than the other, then this locus is the strongest. In parts of Africa pigmentation is fairly uniform, and albinism is both conspicuous and lethal. One locus dominates the scene, and the environment has little contribution to variation. The streets of London offer a wide range of pigmentary variation, but albinos are a rare sight, and not unduly endangered by the strength of the sun. It is clear from the immediate and remote consequences of mixed marriages that many loci are involved, and there is no reason to suppose that the loci most influential in the pigmentary gradients up and down Africa, India and Europe are the same. It is also clear from a study of the beaches of Scandinavia or the airports of Britain that in some areas genetic variation is inconspicuous compared to environmental effects.

In the country of the blind the genetics of sunburn would be as difficult as is the genetics of those other disorders in which a variable threshold of affliction is confounded by a variable exposure to some toxin, irritant or parasite, and concealed by being beneath the skin, or being beyond the resolution of the microscope.

All these associations may be termed "functional", since they relate to similar neighbourhoods on the metabolic map. In order to influence disease manifestation we must shift the mean. For example, dieting reduces the mean weight and, with it, some hazards associated with weight. More subtle population policies, such as the attempt to reduce cholesterol level on a large scale, would seem unwise until evidence on the effects, if any, on other functions, especially intellectual functions, are tested. There seems no indication for genetical advice in the attempt to shift the population mean: indeed, it is not clear why the mean is where it is unless it has got there by selection.

2. *Direct associations due to some determinant influencing the entry of some parasite or toxin into the cell.* Examples include susceptibility to some coliform bacteria in piglets (Rutter *et al.*, 1975), susceptibility of red cells with F_y^a receptors to penetration by some malaria parasites (Miller *et al.*, 1975), and probably the susceptibility of those with the B27 HLA allele to ankylosing spondylitis (Brewerton *et al.*, 1973).

3. *Indirect associations, due to the close linkage, or structural association of a defined locus with another locus.* The predisposition of those with various HLA-B alleles to coeliac disease and diabetes is an example; further studies with a locus known to be closely linked have shown an even stronger association. Both the inferred alleles, and the associated B allele, are different in both these disorders.

We may term these indirect associations "structural", since they are secondary to the nearness of the genetic structures, as opposed to the scene of function of the genetic determinants. In principle some disorders should be both structurally and functionally related: in practice functionally related enzymes seem almost invariably to be defined by structurally unrelated loci.

The HLA System

It has recently been shown that the HLA system, a series of adjoining loci which make the major known contribution within species for defining surface individuality, determine a several-fold range in predisposition to various disorders, varying from a thirty-fold range in ankylosing spondylitis to a ten-fold range in coeliac disease and myasthenia gravis, and somewhat less in diabetes, Hodgkin's disease, and some nasopharyngeal tumours (Möller, 1975).

This should hardly surprise us: to survive we have to take in foodstuffs which nourish us, and we have to coexist both with those species on which we depend for food, and with those which feed on us, especially the bacteria and viruses.

Plants differ from animals in that they cannot run away, and must protect themselves by such other methods as they can contrive. Some plants are prickly, or sting. Others can poison us directly with easily diffusable substances, such as the foxglove which can stop the heart or the poppy which can bemuse the mind. Yet others can attack by exploiting the normal recognition systems at the cell surface, as a result of which they enter in disguise with concealcd arms. Ricin provides a good example: there are two connected molecules, one achieves entry into the cell by fooling the recognition system, the other destroys the cell.

Plants have the same genetic equipment as we have, and, can, and must, match the mobility and intellect of insects, birds and mammals, with an equal wealth of versatility.

So far only wheat, the staple storeable diet of Europe over the last few millennia, has been shown to be toxic to a sufficient minority to be a recognized clinical problem, and some allele, apparently most commonly associated with the 8th allele at the second locus, B8 in the new nomenclature (Bodmer, 1975), exposes its host to an increased risk of irritation to the gut. We may reasonably assume that this is a protective mechanism of the wheat plant which may well have reduced greatly the proportion of persons who were susceptible to it in previous generations.

We can summarize the situation in the plant–mammal system in the simple situation of one-plant and one-mammal. The edible variants will be eaten, leaving those less edible: the mammals will then be reduced by starvation, and by the adverse effects of eating the residual plants, as a result of which the plant population will be restocked by the less digestible survivors. Those mammals able to survive on this fare will then restock the animal numbers, and so the cycle will repeat, with varying cycles of change. Even this simple system provides mathematical problems which give numerical arguments little precision over verbal arguments. When there are many plants and many animals the mathematical problems become insuperable due to the extreme influence of small changes in arbitrary assumptions.

The plant needs to survive, and to outwit our mobility with a range of defensive systems which will match the nervous and locomotor systems of its predators.

The virus, bacteria and other parasites have a similar problem: they must feed on us, but their grazing rights must be defined, otherwise there would be nothing left to graze on. To gain entry, and survive within, they must use similar mechanisms. Further, they must get out again. This vast frontier conflict on the borders of the cell must be conducted with a limited range of weapons, the products of the very similar production lines of all living organisms. In most cases both the primary weapon and the primary defence system are the products of a single locus. Unless we know what we will be eating in the next millennium we would be unwise to attempt to regulate the reproductive habits of those whose recognition systems expose them to the defences of plants and the offences of parasites.

In the last century Olbers pointed out that blackness of the night sky was itself remarkable, for the presence of gaps between stars limited the possibilities of either the stars being unlimited in number, or of the universes being ageless. It is equally remarkable that the ground is green. All around us are mammals, birds and insects, directly or indirectly dependant on leaf protein, and limited in number by starvation in the midst of plenty.

We carry with us our defences from a remote past. If, as seems clear, the crossing-over within the HLA locus is less than 1 per cent, this imposes a half-life of some 2,000 years on the life of any intact segment. Our tissue recognition systems were developed in response to stains of plants we no longer eat, and which may well have disappeared (Fig. 6).

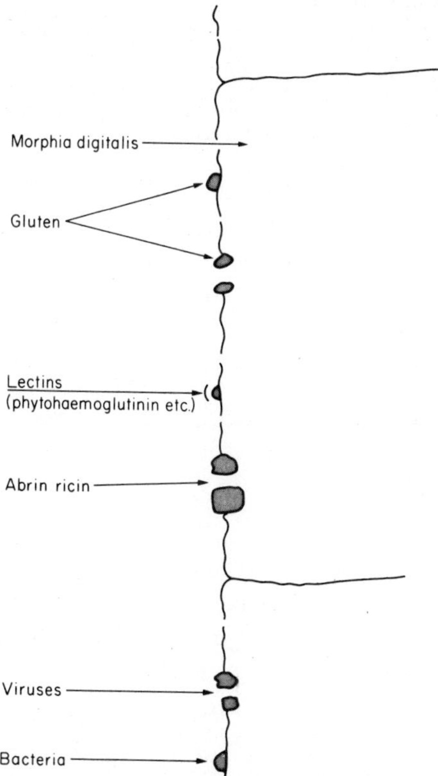

Fig. 6. Showing some ways in which plants defend themselves against man. The cells of the gut have small holes for diffusion of small molecules which are "uncensored" and large ones which are guarded by recognition mechanisms. Other substances can be used as "handholds" for parasites even if they do not enter the cell.

A few, like wheat and rye, still exert a rear-guard action of a few susceptable persons. Some of these systems are an easy prey to some viruses, as is probably the case with ankylosing spondylitis. This is a part of the variability of man which is likely to be quite influential in health and disease as are the chromosome variants which have been disclosed to our gaze by the defensive systems of the runner bean and the autumn crocus.

References

Brewerton, D. A., Caffrey, M., Hart, F. D., James, D. C. O., Nicholls, A. and Sturrock, R. D. (1973). Ankylosing spondylitis and HL-A27. *Lancet*, **i**, 907.

Bodmer, W. F. (1975). Histocompatibility testing international (Review). *Nature*, **256**, 696–698.

Miller, L. H., Mason, S. J., Dvorak, J. A., McGinniss, M. H. and Rothman, I. K. (1975). Erythrocyte receptors for (Plasmodium Knowlesi) malaria: Duffy blood group determinants. *Nature*, **189**, 561.

Möller, G. (Editor) (1975). HL-A and disease. *Transplant Rev*. 22. Copenhagen: Munksgaard.

Rutter, J. F., Burrows, M. R., Sellwood, R. and Gibbons, R. A. (1975). A genetic resistance for binding to enteric disease caused by *E. coli*. *Nature*, **257**, 135.

The Geography of Disease

G. MELVYN HOWE

Department of Geography, University of Strathclyde, Glasgow, Scotland

Disease may be defined as lack of harmony or maladaptation to environmental conditions. Such conditions relate to hazards or stimuli of the physical environment (atmosphere, water, soil), the biological environment (viruses, bacteria and other parasites) and the socio-cultural environment (distribution, density and mobility of populations, nutrition, occupations, housing, habits and customs). The responses to these various stimuli are conditioned by the genetic make-up of the individual. The relative prevalence of the various diseases in the different parts of the world thus reflect differences in the total—physical, biological and socio-cultural—environments and social groups in different geographical areas (Howe, 1972).

In developing countries infectious diseases are still rife and malnutrition and intestinal parasites affect large sections of the population, sapping energy and stunting ability. These are mostly conditions of known origin such as typhoid, cholera, smallpox, rabies, plague, malaria, tuberculosis and kwashiorkor. They could be greatly reduced in frequency and, like smallpox, virtually eliminated if sufficient finance was directed to raising the level of nutrition and sanitation and to implementing necessary programmes of vaccination and control of insect vectors (Oxford Economic Atlas, 1972). With fast and frequent air travel infectious diseases appear occasionally in the economically more prosperous countries within the limit of an incubation period. They are carried by business men and holiday makers and often present diagnostic problems for medical and nursing staff (Bruce-Chwatt, 1974).

In the developed countries infectious diseases have been largely controlled by enlightened environmental changes, health legislation, education and therapeutic advances. The disorders which shorten life in western urbanized and industrialized countries are now of a more

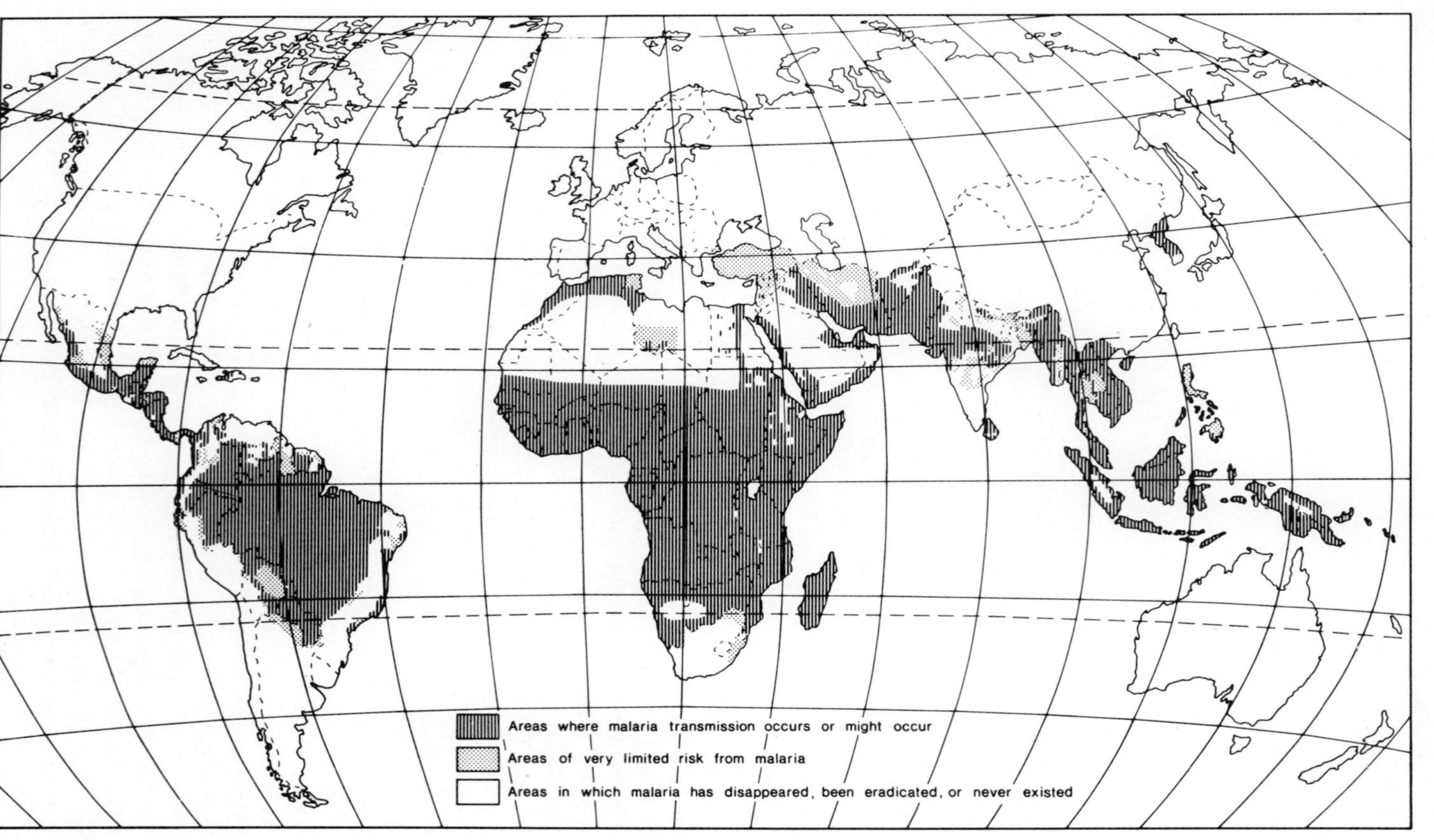

FIG. 1. Malaria (after WHO).

chronic kind. They include diseases of the heart and nervous system (cardiovascular and cerebrovascular diseases), cancer, bronchitis, mental and occupational disorders (Dubos, 1968).

Developing World

Malaria and yellow fever are nowadays restricted to certain tropical regions. The assumptions is that they are "tropical" diseases and yet malaria, for instance, was widespread in temperate lattiudes 100 years ago. Under the name of "ague" malaria was endemic in marshy districts of Britain such as the Fens and East Anglia until the beginning of the twentieth century (Howe, 1972).

The distribution of malaria and its degree of endemicity are closely related to the distribution of the various species of mosquitoes of the genus *Anopheles*. The disease is transmitted to humans through the injection of the sporozoites of the malaria parasite of the genus *Plasmodium*. This takes place when an infected mosquito bites a person (Burnett and White, 1972). Such are the causative circumstances but they do not provide a sufficient condition for the development of malaria. This results only when the exposed person is in a receptive state and this receptivity in its turn affected by the season, the weather and the natural history of the human host—whether, for instance, houses are built on the ground or on piles, whether cooking is done indoors or out, whether domestic animals are kept in or near the house or at a distance, and a host of other ill-defined factors (Fig. 1) (Dubos, 1968).

The progress of the eradication of malaria made in the last three decades has been so phenomenal that ultimate eradication may be in sight. Anopheles mosquitoes do not thrive in urban environments; malaria is thus primarily a disease of the open countryside.

Yellow fever, dengue and dengue haemorrhagic fevers are also mosquito-borne diseases. They are confined to tropical and semi-tropical regions inhabited by the vectors belonging to the sub-genus *Stegomyia* of the genus *Aedes*. At present yellow fever is responsible for recurrent epidemics in Africa and more sporadic infections in South America; it is absent from Asia. The present distribution (Fig. 2) is markedly different from what it was a century ago when severe epidemics of yellow fever recurred throughout the Caribbean area but were not reported from the interior of tropical Africa.

Different from malaria and yellow fever, cholera and influenza spread widely from their point of origin. The form of cholera known as Asiatic is a serious infectious disease. It appears to be endemic in India and China (Fig. 3) but in the nineteenth century there were six major cholera epidemics, several of which swept across Europe and the USA

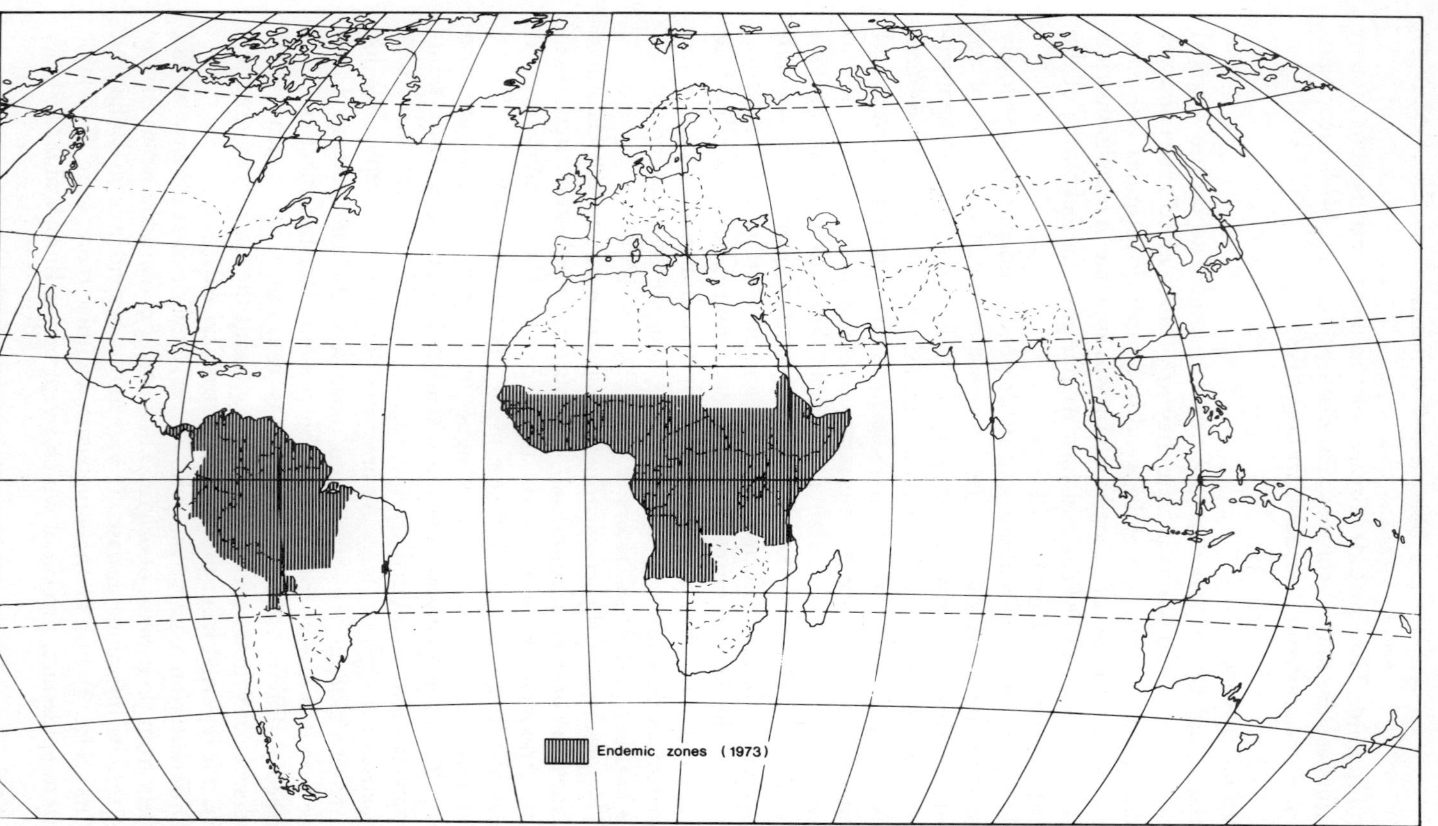

FIG. 2. Yellow fever, endemic zones, 1973 (based on WHO 10920 and WHO 3899).

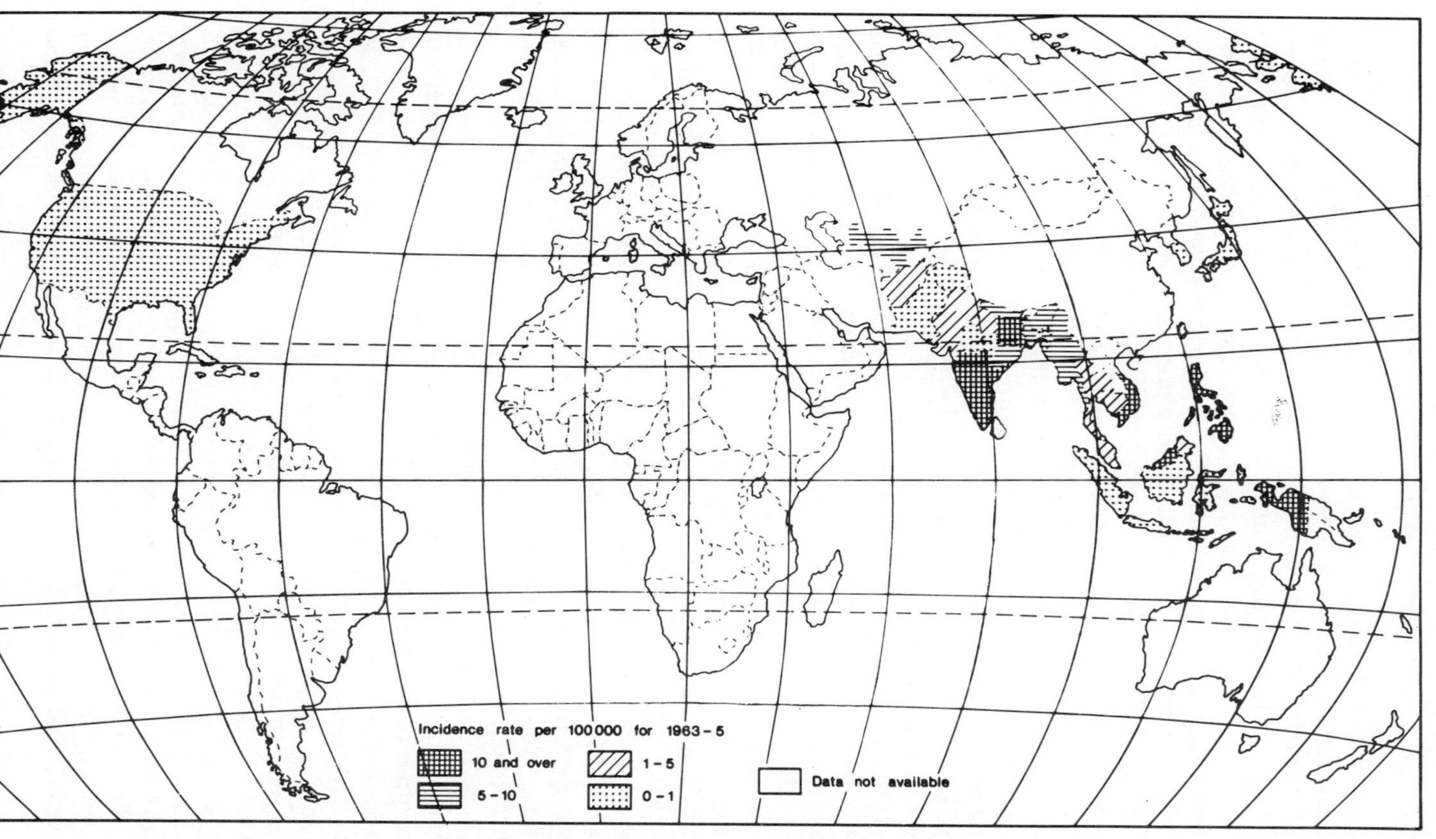

Fig. 3. Asiatic cholera, incidence rates, 1963–65 (after WHO).

as well as the greater part of Asia causing the deaths of millions of people (Longmate, 1966). John Snow, in the mid-nineteenth century, attributed cholera infection to the drinking water contaminated by the excreta of cholera victims (Snow, 1855) but it was not until 1883 that Robert Koch was able to isolate the pathogenic agent, *Vibrio cholerae*. By the 1950s the incidence of cholera in the world appeared to be declining and the disease was thought to be disappearing spontaneously.

Suddenly in 1961 a strain known as cholera *El Tor* started to spread out from a new focus in Sulawezi (the Celebes) in the West Pacific area, South-West Asia, southern European USSR and North Africa. It has since been reported in Spain, Portugal, the Canaries and in West and Central Africa (Fig. 4). It is not known why classical cholera in the nineteenth century of cholera *El Tor* in 1961 relatively suddenly acquired an immense power of dispersion which they have apparently never shown before.

Influenza has travelled around the world more extensively and has been even more pandemic than cholera or the plague. It occurs not only in massive epidemics but also in single cases and sporadically. Its periodicity is irregular; it occurs in all seasons but usually in winter. The disease has been observed in all climatic regions and can affect all races. It is an acute viral disease. Three main influenza viruses, A, B and C, are recognized and classified on the basis of their ribonucleoprotein analysis. The most widespread and most deadly influenza epidemic known to history came in 1918–19 immediately following World War I (Ministry of Health, 1920). In 1968 an epidemic stream of A virus first appeared in the Far East and for four years up to 1972 this so called Hong Kong virus was the prevalent cause of epidemic influenza throughout the world.

Smallpox, possibly the most communicable of all diseases, has been a scourge upon man for untold centuries. There were major epidemics of smallpox in the seventeenth century and it was the most widespread and fatal disease throughout eighteenth century Britain (Howe, 1972). In the nineteenth century, following the work of Edward Jenner, vaccination took the place of variolation and the incidence of smallpox declined. Figure 5 shows the contraction of the endemic countries for smallpox since WHO launched its intensified eradication programme in 1967. In that year the disease was reported in 46 countries, in 1970 in only 14 and in 1971 only nine. In 1975 the only countries reporting smallpox cases are Bangladesh, India and Ethiopia. Total eradication is in sight.

The combination of social progress—improved standard of living, more and better food, better housing, fresh air and sunlight, better hygiene and clean habits—combined with effective chemotherapy has

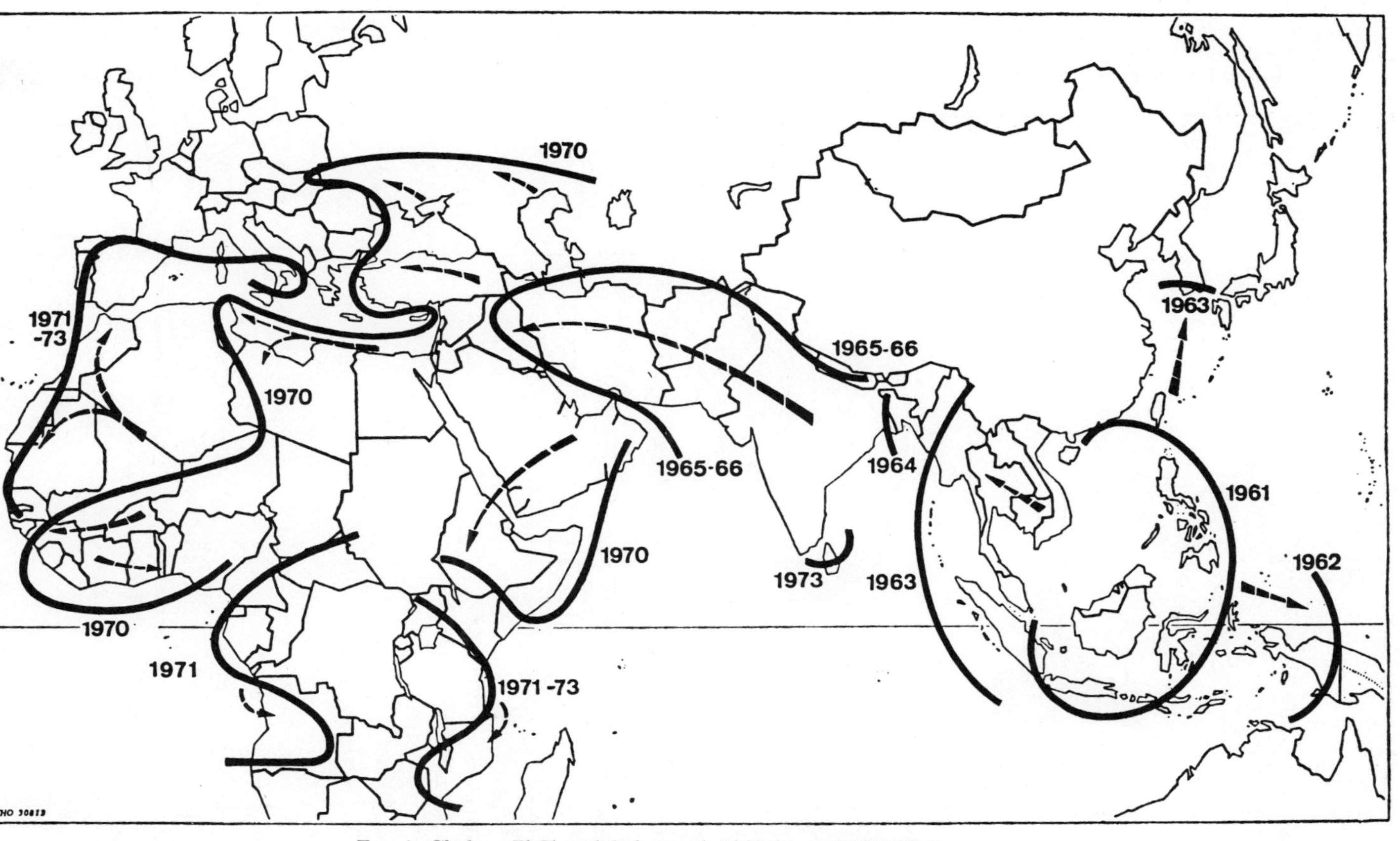

Fig. 4. Cholera *El Tor*; global spread, 1961–73. (WHO 30813).

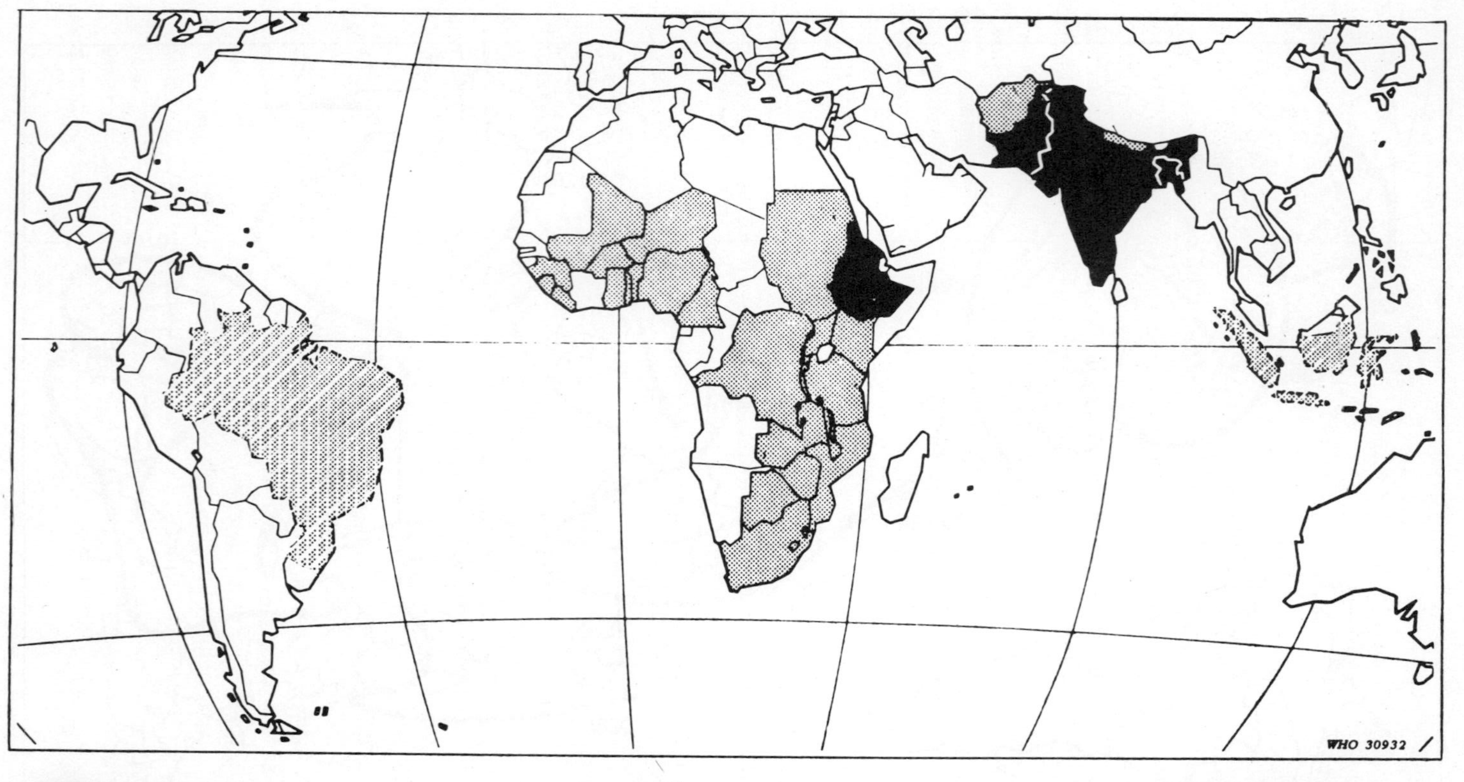

Fig. 5. Smallpox, endemic countries, 1967 and 1974. (WHO 30932).

made tuberculosis relatively unimportant now in the Western world but there is still much to be done in the developing countries with their increasing populations, small budgets and widespread poverty and few facilities for disease control (WHO, 1974) (Fig. 6).

Deficiency diseases are widespread in the developing world (Fig. 7). Their spatial variability makes sense only if they are related to food cultures and when studied as evidence of maladjustment between the society and the environment in which the society lives. Food cultures, in their turn, are a consequence of the soil and climate of the environment and the traditions and economic potential of the human society involved (May, 1961–70). The main deficiency diseases are kwashiorkor (protein malnutrition), marasmus (protein–calorie deficiency), rickets and osteomalacia (calcium and phosphorous or Vitamin D deficiency), goitre and thyroid enlargement and cretinism (iodine deficiency), impaired vision or total blindness (Vitamin A deficiency), beri-beri (deficiency of thiamine), pellagra (niacine deficiency) and scurvy (Vitamin C, ascorbic acid, deficiency).

Developed World

In Western societies, with relatively low birth and death rates and the expectation at birth of a long life ahead, the proportion of people dying from chronic diseases is relatively great.

Cardiovascular disease is now the commonest cause of death in these countries. In Britain ischaemic heart disease is responsible for 25 per cent or nearly 200,000 deaths annually. It affects about four times as many men as women and is most prevalent after the age of 50 years. In developing countries, though little statistical evidence is available, the total mortality from cardiovascular disease is known to be very small, even when allowance is made for the much younger age structure of the population. This fact has given rise to the suggestion of a predisposition to heart disease on the part of white people. Such a hypothesis is belied by the evidence from America where Negroes and Asians have a rate very much higher than is common in most of Africa or India (Fig. 8).

The cause or causes of cardiovascular disease are not known but diets rich in sugar (sucrose), fats or refined carbohydrates (lacking fibre), psychological stress of modern living, obesity, lack of physical exercise, cigarette smoking, high blood pressure and diabetes mellitus are listed as some of the risk factors. Much speculation exists as to the role played by each of these factors and their relative importance (WHO, 1974).

Cancer is second only to cardiovascular disease as a cause of death in the developed world. It is a disease of the cell and affects all races and communities. There are, however, appreciable differences in the fre-

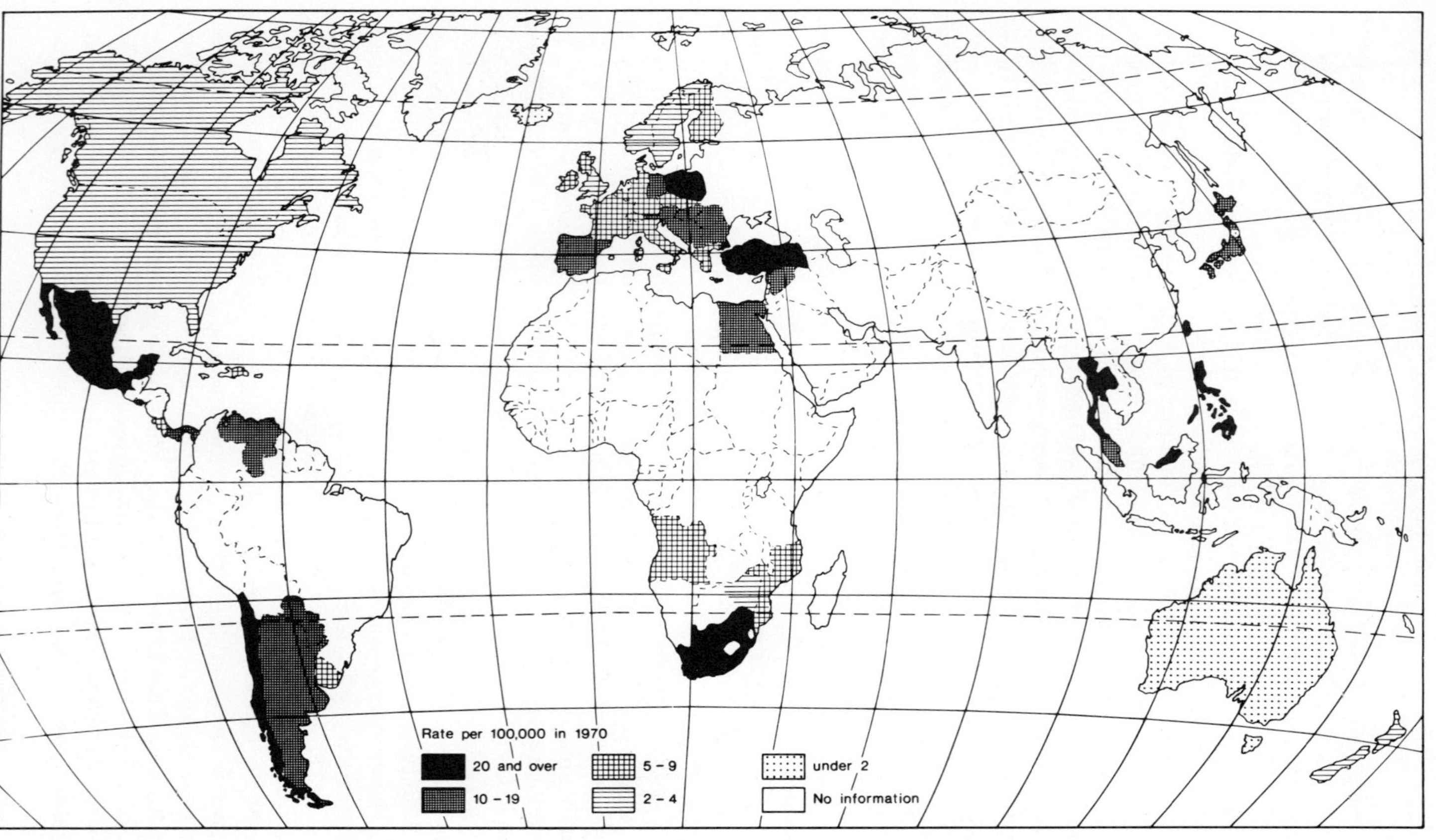

FIG. 6. Tuberculosis, crude rates per 100,000 in 1970 (based on WHO data).

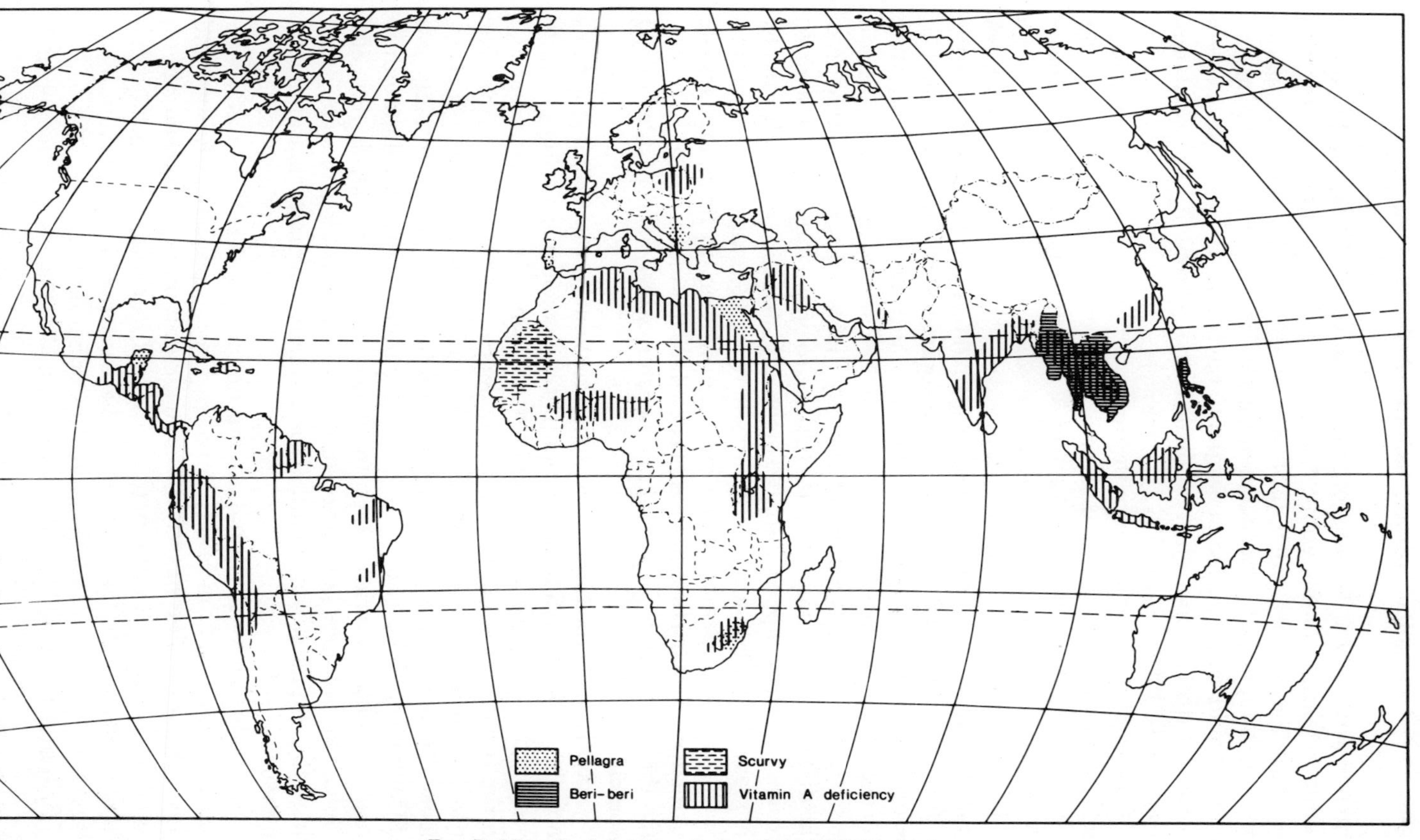

Fig. 7. Vitamin deficiency diseases (after WHO).

quency with which various organs are affected. Thus, while certain common features of malignant disease justify consideration of cancer as an entity, especially when problems at the cellular level are under investigation, nonetheless cancer of each individual organ in the human body should be regarded separately. Each has its own distinct geographical distribution when studied at the community or population level (Doll, 1969; Howe, 1972).

Cancer of the liver and mouth are more frequent in southern Africa and India than in Europe or North America. The reverse is true for cancer of the large intestine. Cancer of the lung and bronchus appears to be more common in Britain than anywhere else in the world, though it is also widespread in central and eastern Europe, USSR and USA (Fig. 9). Incidence is slightly less in Canada, Australia and among the white population of South Africa, and considerably less in Scandinavia, South America and Asia. It is virtually unknown in East and West Africa but among Africans in the towns of Zambia and South Africa it has become one of the more commonly diagnosed tumours. Wherever the disease is now common it has become so only within the last 30 or 40 years and there appears to be mounting evidence to implicate the increase in cigarette smoking. Everywhere the increase in lung-bronchus cancer has been greater among men than women. In Britain the female incidence has started to increase faster than the male, probably reflecting the time-lag before smoking became widely acceptable among women.

Japan records the highest incidence of stomach cancer but it is common throughout Soviet Asia. From there the incidence declines steadily westwards to a much lower level in North America. The one exception to the trend is Iceland where the incidence is unexpectedly high. The distribution is less regular in the southern hemisphere (Fig. 10). Incidence is generally low in Africa although there are some areas, e.g. east of Congo Republic, where it is the most commonly diagnosed tumour in men. In South America a high incidence is recorded in Colombia and Chile. The Japanese population of Hawaii have far less stomach cancer than the Japanese in Japan. This strongly suggests environmental influences.

Stomach cancer is unusual among tumours in that there has been a general reduction in mortality in recent years, especially in Europe and North America. This has led to the suggestion that carcinogenic agents could be produced by the deterioration of foodstuffs, which has been largely checked in the West with the widespread introduction of refrigeration and better methods of food preservation.

Brittany, Curacao, Jamaica and Malawi are known to have a high

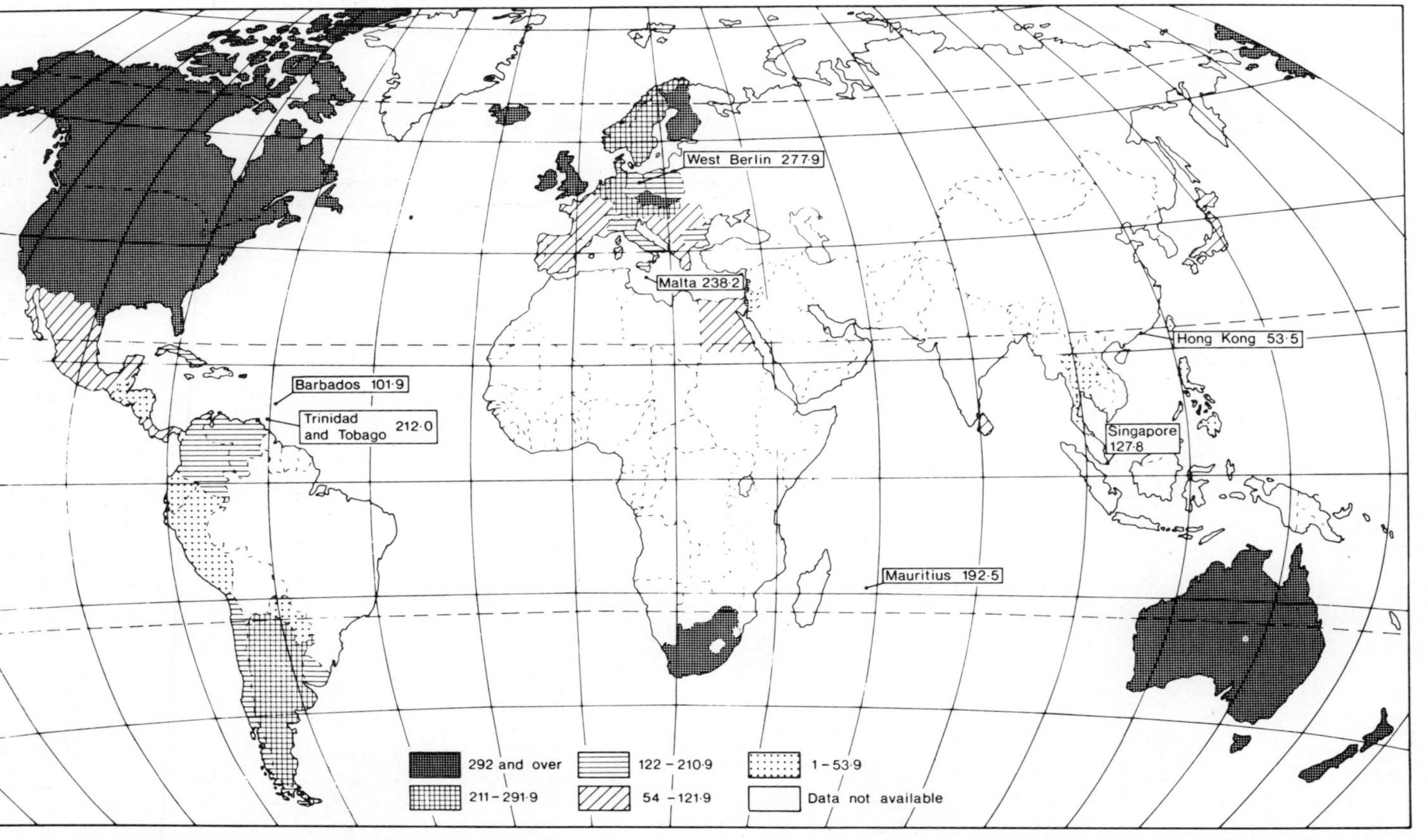

FIG. 8. Ischaemic heart disease, average annual age—standardized mortality rates, 35-64 years, males, 1969–71 (based on WHO data).

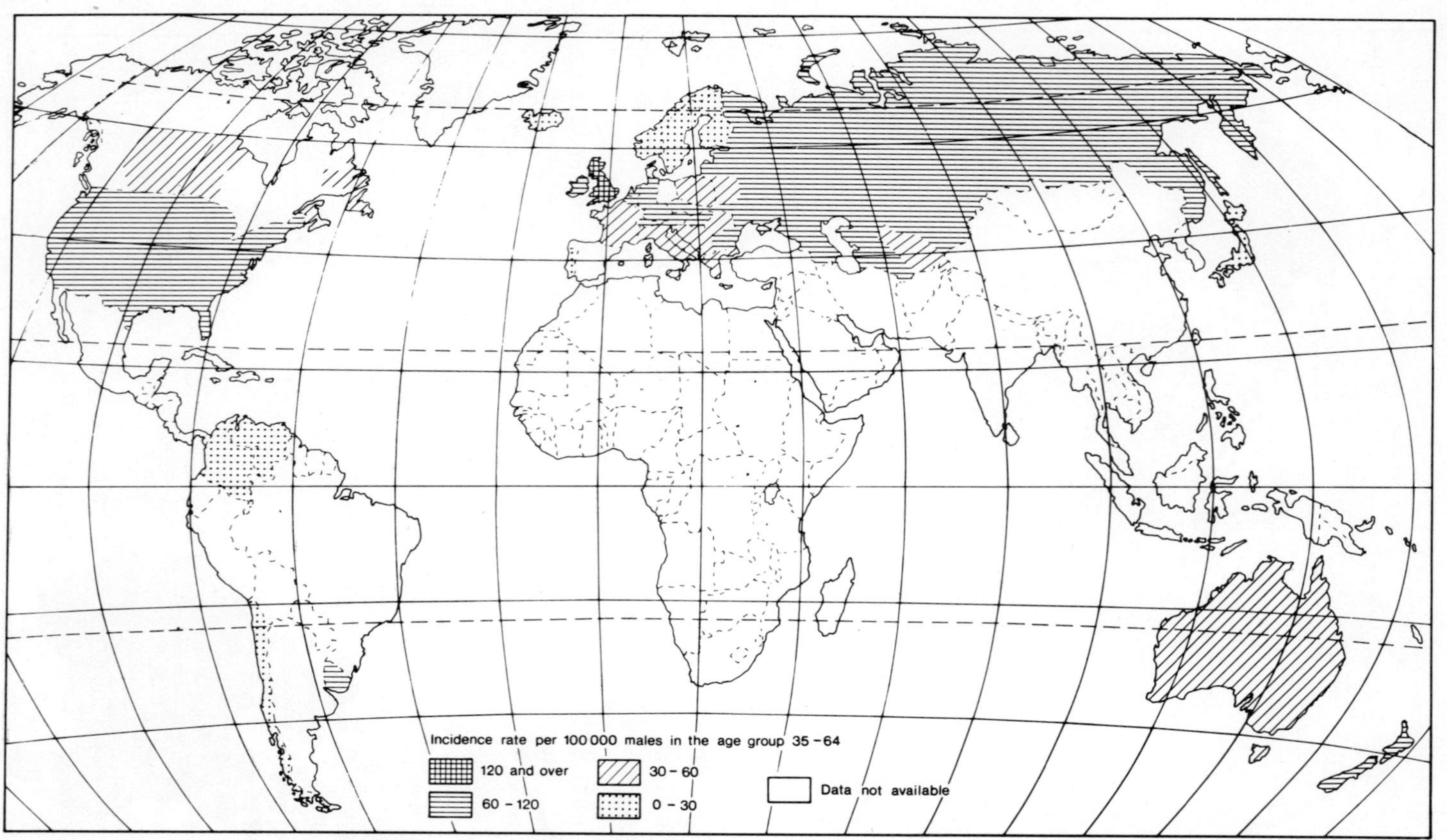

Fig. 9. Lung cancer, incidence rate per 100,000 males, in 35–64 years age group (based on WHO data).

incidence of oesophageal cancer. The common link is a certain liking people of these regions share for their local alcoholic beverages or, in the case of Curacao, their hot maize porridge. The northern coast of Iran along the Caspian has three regions with different climates and life patterns and different patterns of oesophageal cancer. Clues to date have tended to implicate trace elements (Willard, 1970).

The most striking feature of the regional distribution of chronic bronchitis is that the mortality in the UK is about thirty times greater than in the USA and five or six times greater than in most of western Europe (Fig. 11). Within Britain it is a town disease. It appears to correlate with heavily industrialized and polluted areas; rural areas with slight air pollution seem to escape. Bronchitis is also a disease of the poor. Mortality is highest among unskilled men and women, the rate falling progressively to the lowest among professional men and women (Howe, 1972).

The study of global variations in the distributions of mental disorders and mental subnormality is a comparatively new phenomenon and fraught with difficulties related to the fundamental problems of definition. The calculated act of self destruction, suicide, is a specifically human behavioural attribute (Fig. 12). Between 1964 and 1966 suicide was among the first ten causes of death in 21 industrialized countries and one of the ten leading causes of death in 33 countries for persons in the age group 15–44 years. In Austria, Denmark, the Federal German Republic, Hungary, Sweden and Switzerland suicide ranked third after cancer and coronary heart disease for this age group. Evidence would suggest that national suicide rates reflect significant variations in national characteristics. For example, a study of suicide rates among immigrants from 11 countries into the USA revealed that they were virtually identical with those recorded in the countries from which they had emigrated (Tredgold and Soddy, 1970; Lynn, 1971).

Since about the early 1960s incidence of those conditions known internationally as sexually-transmitted diseases (STD) has started to rise. STDs now comprise the largest single category of communicable diseases in the world, on a par with the common cold.

The above severely restricted selection of human diseases demonstrates the appreciable spatial variability of disease incidence and disease mortality throughout the world. The distribution reflect ecological imbalance in different parts of the world and, since man is radically changing the ecology of life on this planet, disease patterns are dynamic. From the health point of view, some of the changes may be good, some may be harmful and others may prove catastrophic. The possible proliferation of nuclear weapons and heavy future dependence on nuclear

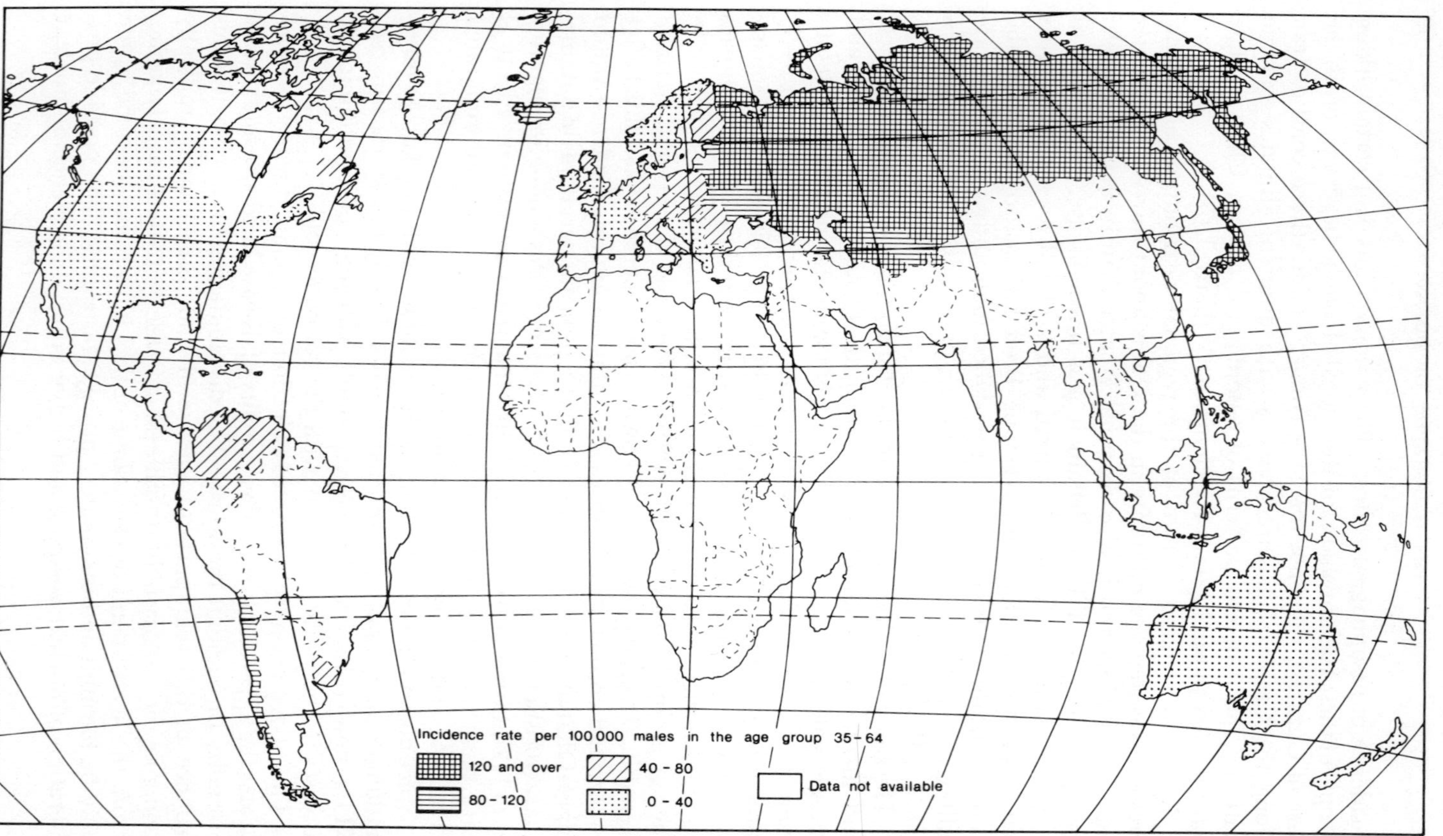

FIG. 10. Stomach cancer, incidence rate per 100,000 males in 35–64 years age group (based on WHO data).

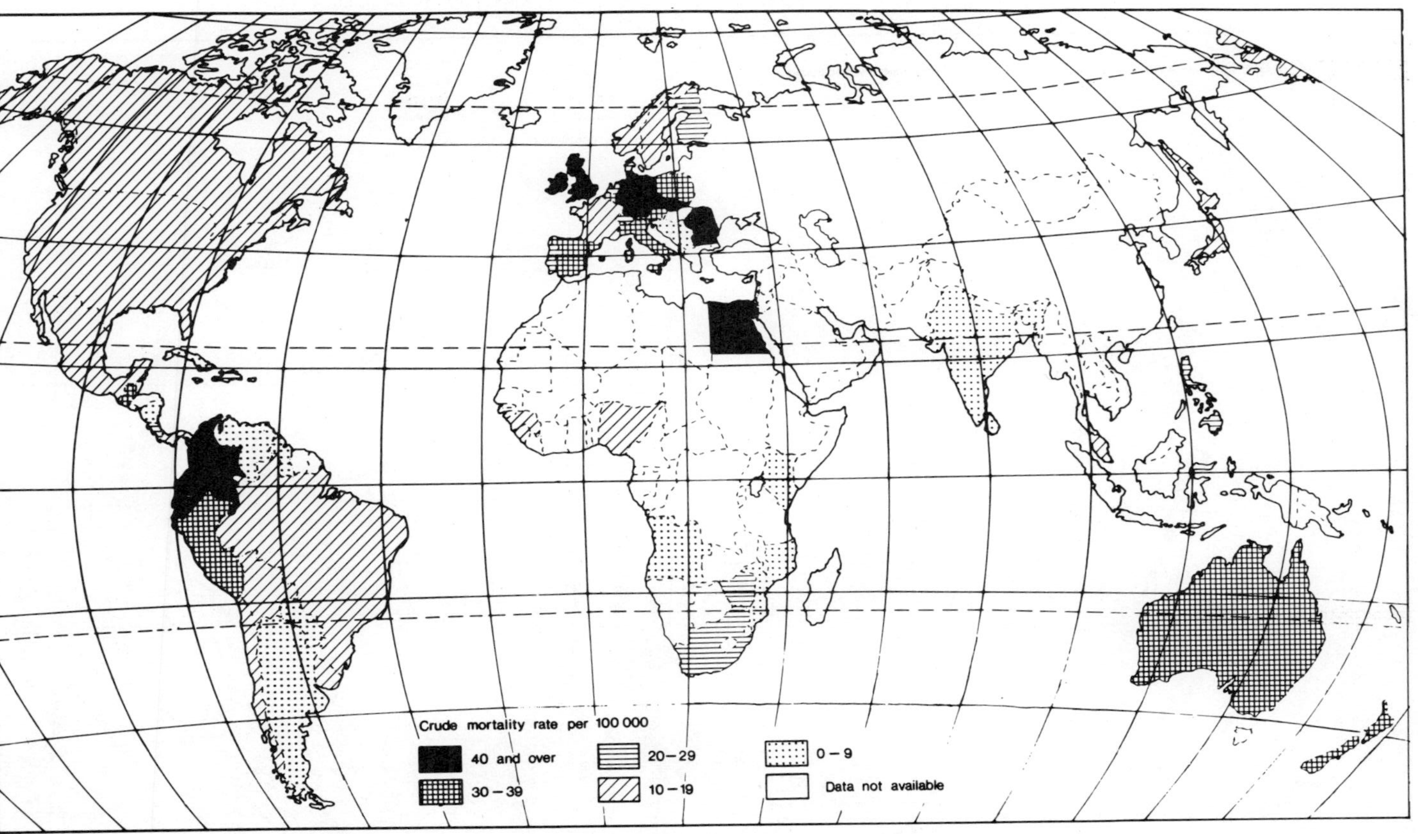

Fig. 11. Bronchitis, crude mortality rates—both sexes (based on UN Demographic Year-book, 1970).

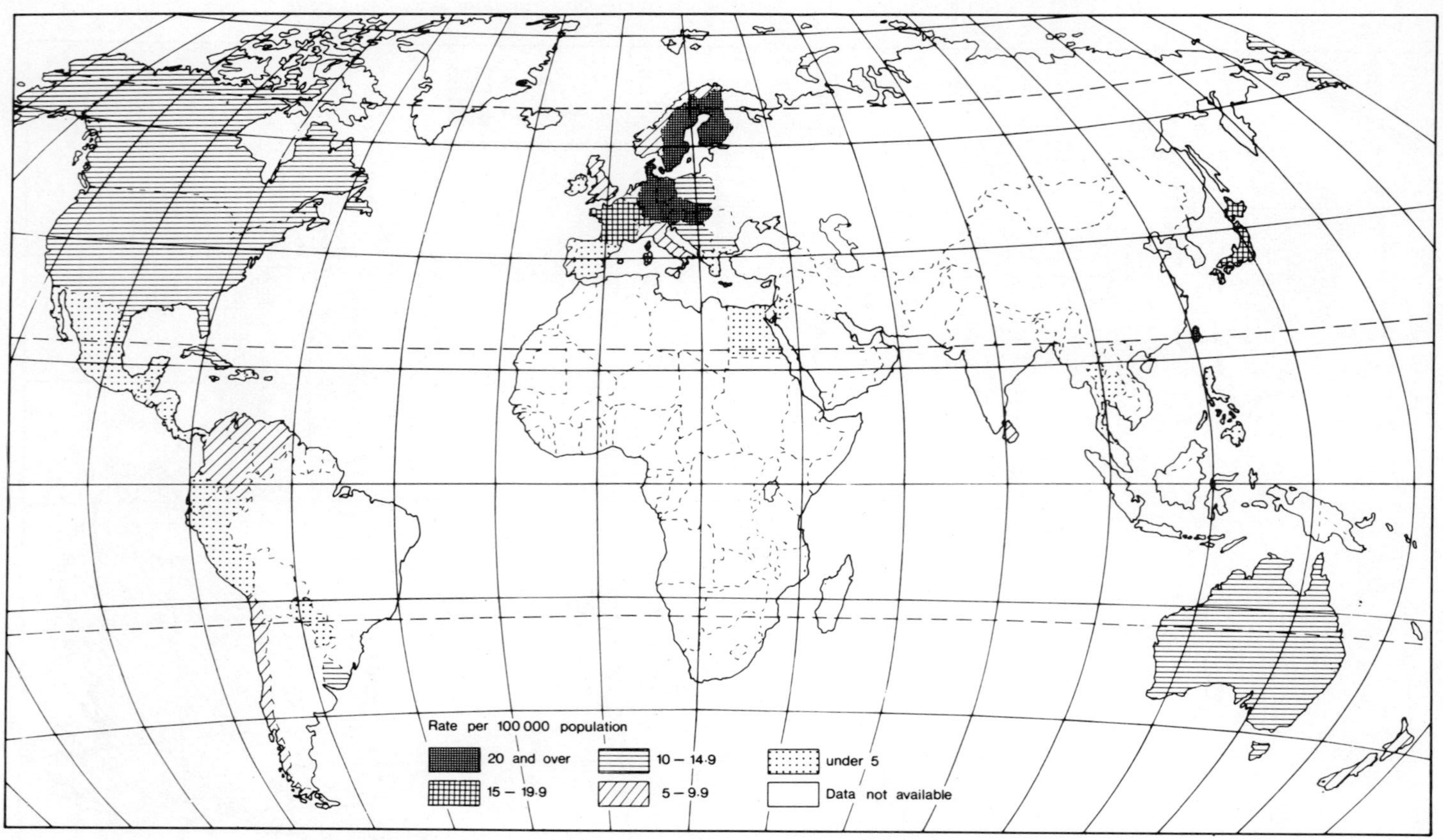

Fig. 12. Suicide, crude mortality rates (based on WHO Statistical Reports, 1972 and 1973).

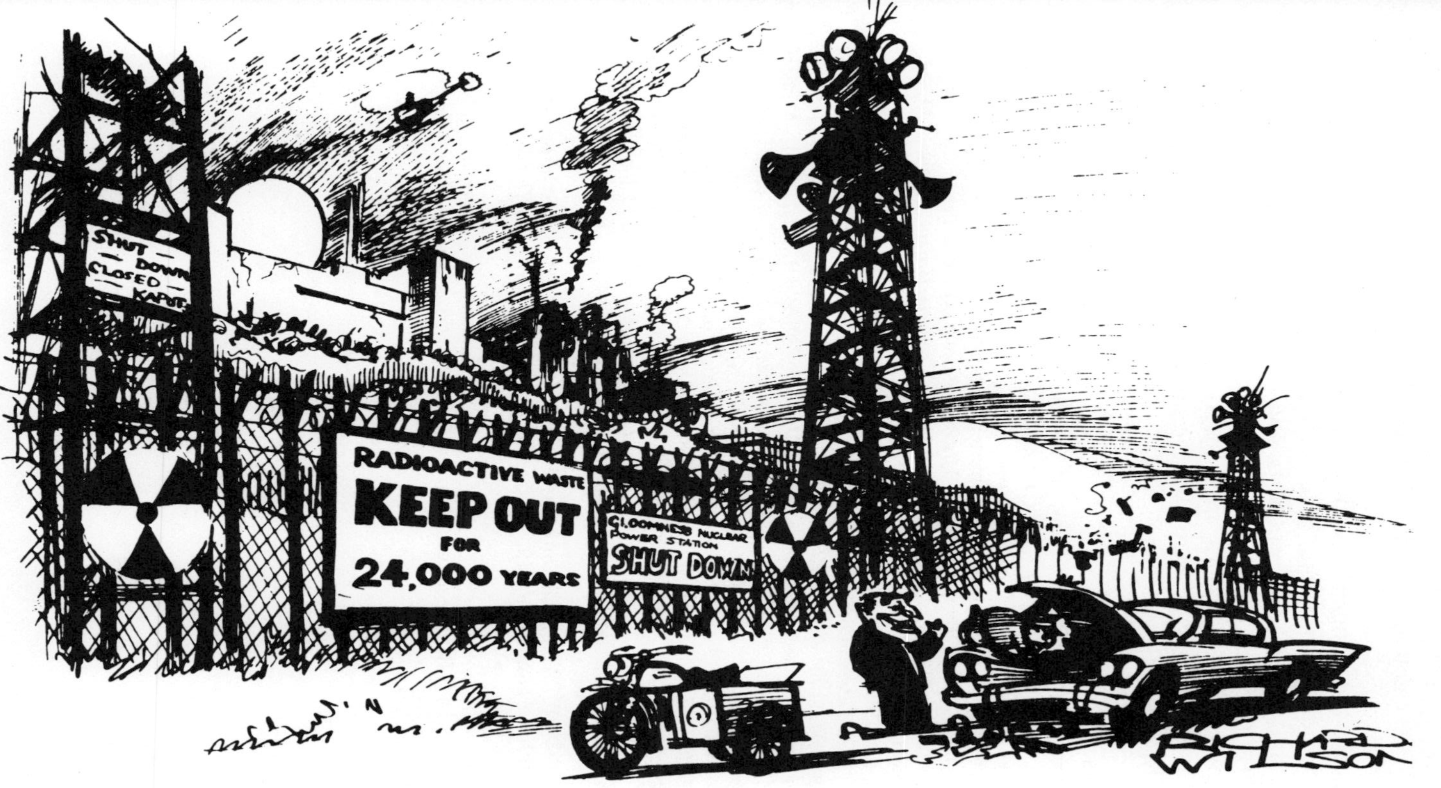

FIG. 13. The danger of radioactive waste: with acknowledgements to the *New Scientist*.

energy poses the danger of highly dangerous radioactive fallout and long-lived radioactive wastes (Fig. 13). Foolproof reactors are not yet available and an accident would be the most decisive of all events in human history, from the point of view of both environmental change and predisposition to disease in man. It would be a tragedy if "the sunrise of technology were to be the sunset of mankind" (Winston Churchill).

References

Bruce-Chwatt, L. J. (1974). Air transport and disease. *J. Biosoc. Sci.*, **6**, 241–258.

Burnett, M. and White, D. O. (1972). *Natural History of Infectious Disease.* 4th ed. Cambridge: Cambridge University Press.

Doll, R. (1969). The geographical distribution of cancer. *Br. J. Cancer* **23**, 1–18.

Dubos, R. (1968). *Man, Environment and Medicine.* New York: Praeger.

Howe, G. Melvyn (1972). *Man, Environment and Disease in Britain.* Newton Abbot: David and Charles.

Longmate, N. (1966). *King Cholera. The Biography of a Disease.* London: H. Hamilton.

Lynn, R. (1971). Personality and National Character. Oxford: Pergamon.

May, Jacques M. (1961–70). *The Ecology of Malnutrition in: the Far and Near East* (1961); *Five Countries of Eastern and Central Europe* (1963); *Middle Africa* (1965); *Northern Africa* (1967); *French speaking Countries of West Africa and Madagascar* (1968); *Eastern Africa and Four Countries of Western Africa* (1970). New York: Hafner.

Ministry of Health (1920). Report on the pandemic of influenza 1918–19. *Report Public Health and Medical Subjects No. 4*, London: Her Majesty's Stationery Office.

Oxford Economic Atlas of the World (1972). 4th ed. Oxford University Press.

Tredgold, R. F. and Soddy, K. (1970). *Tredgold's Mental Retardation.* 11th ed. London.

Snow, J. (1855). *On the Mode of Communication of Cholera.* 2nd ed. London: Bailliere Tindall.

Willard, N. (1970). The riddle of many regions. *Wld Hlth* Feb.–March, pp. 14–19.

World Health Organization (1974). Cardiovascular diseases. *WHO Chronicle* **28**, 55–64, 116–125.

World Health Organization (1974). *WHO Expert Committee on Tuberculosis.* Ninth Report. World Health Technical Report Series No. 552. London: Her Majesty's Stationery Office.

The Assessment of Risks to Health at Work

W. R. LEE

Department of Occupational Health,
University of Manchester, Oxford Road, Manchester, England

> Everyone is in favour of purposes beneficial to the community, but if everyone agreed what they were, politicians would cease to exist.
>
> (*The Times*, 1975)

Introduction

There is a great deal of interest at the present time in our environment and its possible effects on the population. For many years, occupational medicine has provided a unique opportunity for study in this field. In industry, we are frequently able to describe not only the environment with some degree of accuracy, both with regard to its constituents and to the concentrations of these constituents, but also we have, at the same time, a population of exposed persons which is generally well defined and which may be under medical surveillance. This medical surveillance may be designed to monitor the expected specific effects on the population of one or more identified constituents of the environment. For example, we might study pulmonary function in asbestos workers, or the metabolites of chlorinated hydrocarbons in the urine of persons exposed to trichlorethylene or related solvents.

As a result of these observations, the environment may be changed; either the general environment or the personal micro-environment of the worker, so that those changes which we do detect in him are not harmful. This statement implies that a decision has been reached about the level of change in the working environment which may be considered harmful. It also implies that a mechanism has been evolved for reaching such a decision. It is these two matters which I wish to discuss today—firstly, the principles on which a decision is reached that a particular working environment is acceptable. Secondly, the administrative machinery which has evolved and which might be developed for reaching these decisions.

Principles Regulating Decisions

When referring to an abstract idea such as decision making, I have used the words "mechanism" and "machinery", and it is interesting to reflect how, over the last two centuries, such "mechanical" metaphors have entered our language. Not only have the metaphors entered our language, but the concepts of mechanical engineering often seem subconsciously to influence our approach to problems. Thus, walking through almost any factory, we notice that ladders, cranes and similar devices have painted on the side the letters S.W.L. for Safe Working Load. This implies that so long as that particular crane or ladder is not loaded above the stated figure it will not collapse—and, customarily, the engineer has added a generous safety factor in his calculations. It is not surprising, therefore, that occupational medicine has followed this lead by defining the permissible working environment in terms such as Threshold Limit Value and Maximum Allowable Concentration. Such terms have the natural, if perhaps unwarranted, implication that we are "safe" so long as we keep below the "threshold", or so long as we do not exceed the allowable maximum.

However, we have increasingly come to realize when studying the effects of the working environment on groups of exposed workers, that we are dealing not so much with a clearly defined boundary as with a situation of probability. Let me give two examples. The International Commission on Radiological Protection stated in 1959:

> Any departure from the environmental conditions in which man has evolved, may entail a risk of deleterious effects. It is, therefore, assumed that long continued exposure to ionizing radiation additional to that due to natural radiation involves some risk. However, man cannot entirely dispense with the use of ionizing radiation and, therefore, the problem in practice is to limit the radiation dose to that which involves a risk that is not unacceptable to the individual and to the population at large.

A few years later, the United Nations Scientific Committee on the Effects of Atomic Radiation (1964) calculated the rate of increase of leukaemia, which is considered the major component of the total risk from radiation exposure, with increasing dose. They presumed a linear dose response relationship at low doses and decided that the rate of increase of leukaemia was about 1 to 2 cases per yard per rad per million persons irradiated for ten years.

To take another example, in a report on asbestosis from chrysotile (white) asbestos dust, the Committee of Hygiene Standards of the British Occupational Hygiene Society (Lane *et al.*, 1968) concluded that:

> As long as there is an appreciable amount of dust in the air, the Committee recognises that there may be some risk to health.

After reviewing the available evidence linking known exposure to chrysotile dust with the occurrence of the earliest detectable changes of asbestosis, whether clinical or radiological, they calculated that the risk of developing asbestosis is about one per cent for workers exposed to a concentration of 2 fibres per cm^3 over a working lifetime of 50 years. This recommendation, like the one for radiation just cited, does not refer to a safe level but specifies the risk.

These are examples and there are others, that we are faced, not with a definable boundary between safe and hazardous, but with a zone of uncertainty. As we move into this zone of uncertainty, we can describe our position by referring to a changing probability of an effect being produced. In fact, we may be able to determine, with some degree of accuracy, the relative position of two points in this zone of uncertainty by observing the relative probabilities of groups of exposed persons being affected, or, alternatively, by observing the changing incidence of harmful effects detectable in the two groups.

I do not wish to repeat the comparisons between risks at work and risks at recreation which have been made elsewhere (Sowby, 1965; Pochin, 1973). As Cohen (1964) has pointed out:

> The degree of uncertainty we tolerate in everyday life, like the risks and hazards we incur at home or at work, change in a curious fashion when we enter the world of play.

I think it is necessary to accept that we have a stochastic situation and to consider what guides we should use to govern our decisions on the amounts of certain materials to which workpeople may be exposed. Before we do so, it is useful to realize that we are by no means alone in this predicament. It is more than 40 years since Heisenberg was awarded the Nobel Prize in Physics for his Principle of Indeterminacy. He wrote:

> The electrons which form the shells in an atom are no longer things in the sense of classical physics, things which could be unambiguously described by concepts like location, velocity, energy, size. When we get down to the atomic level, the objective world in space and time no longer exists, and the mathematical symbols of theoretical physics refer merely to possibilities, not to facts.

The Principle of Indeterminacy put an end to causal determinism, not only in physics but also in philosophy (Koestler, 1974). A telling example is given by Magee (1973) from Karl Popper on the measurement of length. You can only get a piece of steel *approximately* six millimetres long. The very best instruments may make it to a degree of accuracy within a millionth of a millimetre, but where, within that margin, lies the exact point of six millimetres we cannot, in the nature of things, know. Popper goes on to maintain the essential feature of a law of science is not its inviolability but its falsibility. Such laws do not prescribe events but only describe them.

Whatever the impact of recent developments in uncertainty on the philosophy of science, it has long been recognized in moral philosophy, that the answers to ethical questions can be neither logically demonstrated nor experimentally verified (Joad, 1938). One famous attempt to meet this dilemma is the greatest happiness principle associated with Jeremy Bentham, that morality consists in obtaining the maximum amount of happiness for the greatest number of people. This was developed by John Stuart Mill who sought to differentiate quality of pleasure as well as quantity of pleasure. Furthermore, Mill was not content with "happiness" as a concept but modified it to "the greatest benefit", denoting the experience of health among the achievement of such beneficial experiences (Campbell, 1972).

There have been many criticisms of the theory of greatest happiness. Foremost amongst these are the practical difficulties of defining happiness (or benefit) and of predicting happiness (or benefit) (Campbell, 1972). To this one might add the question, "In what units is the calculation of greatest happiness or greatest benefit to be made?" This is not academic speculation for already in the modern application of Mill's principles the unit of calculation used is the unit of currency. Such are "cost benefit analysis" and "total loss control".

The idea that human life should be regarded as anything but sacred is foreign to medicine, for within our Western society and maybe in others, the medical ethic includes the sanctity of life. Indeed, the phrase "the sanctity of life" implies that life is "holy" and reflects the depth that religion penetrates the thought of our culture. Nevertheless, money is almost generally used at the present time as the unit in calculations of greatest benefit, even where life may be concerned.

To take an example from a related field, Hayzelden (1968), in a thoughtful paper on "The Value of Human Life", accepted that "value" might be measured in money and began by considering the question "The value to whom?" His paper dealt with public administration and he rejected as not relevant in his context the question "What has X lost when he dies?" and "What have X's dependants lost?" He suggested that the real question, to the public administrator was "What has society lost when X dies?" As an example, he took the construction of an underpass at a road junction, using the financial terms of 1968. This might cost an annual £0·6m and the estimated annual benefit (in reduced traffic congestion, etc.) would be £0·5m + 5 lives saved. If each life was valued at £25,000, the project would be financially worthwhile; if at £15,000 it would not. One advantage of that example is that it only makes the simple contrast between human life and its value to society. The problem is not complicated by the question of employment and by the introduction of a third element such as shareholders, but we shall shortly need to take that into our considerations.

Means of Arriving at Decisions

We are now, therefore, in a situation where "the greatest benefit" model of Bentham and Mill is generally used to regulate our affairs, but that the only units in which we may attempt to calculate this "greatest benefit" are financial. Although we may have to accept this, many will have reservations when attempts are made to measure in financial terms factors which they consider as immeasurable.

The next step is to ask, "Who should do those calculations and make the decisions based on them?" Because the units are financial there may be a temptation to leave the decisions to cost accountants. But, there are two things to be borne in mind—firstly, some of the factors are not readily measured and, secondly, as noted earlier, we are often concerned with assessing probabilities rather than working with thresholds. We may reduce the probability from 1 in 100 to 1 in 10,000 but we cannot say which of the exposed persons will be affected. Furthermore, it is not a simple two sided calculation of the benefits to society on the one hand, measured against the unhappiness of reduced benefit of one or more individuals on the other. Where there is a private sector of industry there is introduced a third element of the shareholders representing their own interests and perhaps the existence or even the viability of the enterprise itself, and to some extent, therefore, the interests of society as a whole. There are three parties, then, who are interested in our calculation of greatest benefit. They are industry (represented by management), the work-people, and society or the general public. I think that this would be true if units other than money were used for the calculations.

How are these three groups to contribute to the decision on greatest benefit? Before we consider this question for the future, it is relevant to note that, although these problems may have become more prominent, they are not suddenly new. It is, therefore, useful to look at the methods which have evolved by which such problems have been dealt with up to the present time.

We permit people to work in an atmosphere containing 100 parts per million of toluene but only 10 parts per million of benzene. How were these figures arrived at, and by whom? They were arrived at after careful consideration of the scientific evidence, both clinical observations on humans, and experimental studies with animals. They were proposed by an American scientific body of high repute, the American Conference of Governmental and Industrial Hygienists, and the figures have been copied, presumably after due scrutiny, by our Department of Labour, now the Health and Safety Executive. The determination of such values, although not necessarily the values themselves, has been challenged by the American Labour Unions as "scientific meeting in secret conclave". Perhaps this is a reaction against the composition of the standard setting body in that it did not represent the three groups of management, workers and society, mentioned above. It illustrates the point that health and safety standards are more likely to be acceptable to those who must comply with them if they are conceived as "our" standard, rather than "theirs". Similarly, the authors of the widely accepted British Hygiene Standard for protection against chrysotile asbestos dust, discussed earlier, are all prominent doctors and scientists.

Another example is protection against radiation. The International Commission on Radiological Protection has recommended standards for many years, and experts from this country have contributed to the discussions (1959). In Britain, the National Radiological Protection Board (NRPB) is responsible for investigating and advising on radiological protection. It is an autonomous scientific body set up by the government.

However, decisions on health and safety standards have generally been made in this country by one of the government inspectorates, customarily the Factory Inspectorate. These functions have recently been taken over by the Health and Safety Executive. In exercising these functions, such government bodies consult management and the trades unions, but the ultimate decision rests with the Health and Safety Executive (HSE).

This leads to the question whether one body should combine both legislation and enforcement functions. More baldly, should the policeman make the laws which he enforces?

We have already seen that there is a precedent in this country for the separation for radiological protection of standard setting (National Radiological Protection Board) from enforcement (Health and Safety Executive). In America also, recent legislation has divided, in this instance into separate government departments, the function of standard setting on the one hand, by the National Institute for Occupational Safety and Health (NIOSH), from enforcement on the other by the Occupational Safety and Health Administration (Table I). Admittedly, in neither of these examples does the standard setting body (NRPB and NIOSH) comprise the three groups of management, workers and general public, which I have reasoned is desirable. The point here is the separation of the legislative, or standard setting, function from the executive function.

TABLE I

Separation of legislative and enforcement functions

	Legislative/Enforcement	
	Standard setting	Enforcement
UK	National Radiological Protection Board	Health and Safety Executive
USA	National Institute of Occupational Health and Safety	Occupational Safety and Health Administration

If we accept then that there should be a standard setting organization, that it should contain the three groups already mentioned and that it should be separate from the enforcement function, where might it be set?

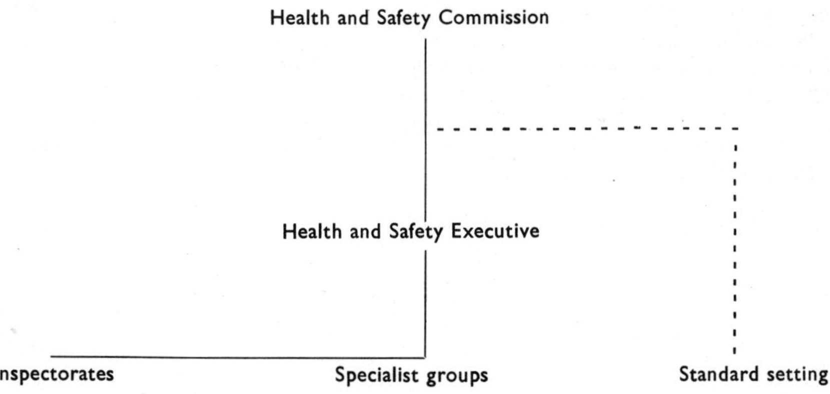

FIG. 1. Proposed relationship of standard setting body.

Under the new Health and Safety at Work Act, there is already established the Health and Safety Commission which oversees the duties of the Health and Safety Executive and comprises representatives of the CBI, TUC and Local Authorities. It would not be difficult to envisage a standard setting body within this Health and Safety Commission, with the composition and functions proposed in this lecture, which is separate from the Health and Safety Executive with its enforcement functions but advisory to the Commission (Fig. 1).

In this way, we could recognize that in our participating society where there is an increasing number of these matters to be considered, the views of all those who are most affected are represented, the decisions will be more likely to attract wide support.

References

Campbell, A. V. (1972). *Moral Dilemmas in Medicines*, pp. 51, 57. London: Churchill Livingstone.

Cohen, J. (1964). *Behaviour in Uncertainty*, p. 118. London: George Allen and Unwin.

Hayzelden, J. E. (1968). The value of human life. *Public Admin.* **46**, 427–442.

Heisenberg, W. (1969). Cited by A. Koestler (1974) in *The Roots of Coincidence*, p. 51. London: Picador Books.

Joad, C. E. M. (1938). *Guide to the Philosophy of Morals and Politics*, p. 148. London: Victor Gollancz.

Koestler, A. (1974). *The Roots of Coincidence*, p. 51. London: Picador Books.

Lane, R. E., Barnes, J. M., Hichins, D. E., Jones, A. G., Roach, S. A. and King, E. (1968). Hygiene standards for chrysotile asbestos dust. *Ann. Occ. Hyg.* **11**, 47–69.

Magee, B. (1973). *Popper*, p. 27. London: Fontana/Collins.

Pochin, E. E. (1973). Levels of hazard in various occupations. In *The Assessment of Exposure and Risk*. Edited by B. W. Duch, pp. 33–58. London: Society of Occupational Medicine, Royal College of Physicians.

Recommendations of the International Commission on Radiological Protection. (1959). Oxford: Pergamon Press.

Sowby, F. D. (1965). Radiations and other risks. *Hlth Phys.* **11**, 879–887.

The Times. (1975). Leading Article. 26th September.

United Nations Scientific Committee on the Effects of Atomic Radiation. (1964). *Report to the General Assembly*. General Assembly Document Suppl. No. 14. (A/5814). Geneva: United Nations.

The Galton Lecture: 1975

Inequality: Is It Inevitable?

SIR JOHN BROTHERSTON

Scottish Home and Health Department, Scotland

Social Class Differences in Mortality and Morbidity

There is so much evidence demonstrating differences in mortality and morbidity between the social classes as defined by our Registrars General that it is difficult to select from the evidence. These differences are well known. I demonstrate them here in terms of total mortality experience for adults. I demonstrate also differences in experience in maternity and infancy—the maternal mortality rate is demonstrated but today the perinatal mortality rate is a better measure of different experience in obstetrics.

TABLE I

Male standardized mortality ratios: by social class England and Wales

	1921–23) (age 20–64	1930–32 (age 20–64)	1949–53 (age 20–64)	1959–63 (age 15–64)	1970–72* (age 15–64)
Social class					
I	82	90	86	76	77
II	94	94	92	81	81
III	95	97	101	100	104
IV	101	102	104	103	113
V	125	111	118	143	137

From Central Statistical Office (1975).
The Table Sources are marked as 1921–63 RGs Decennial Supplements: Occupation Mortality 1951 and 1961 1970–72 Office of Population Census and Surveys.
* i.e. the 1970–72 figures are marked "Provisional data".

TABLE II

Infant mortality rates per 1,000 live births by social class for Scotland 1961 and 1970

Social class	1961	1970	Per cent decrease 1961–70
I and II	17·4	12·0	31
III	25·1	18·6	26
IV and V	30·0	25·4	15
IV and V as a percentage of I and II	172·0	212·0	

From Scottish Register General's Data.

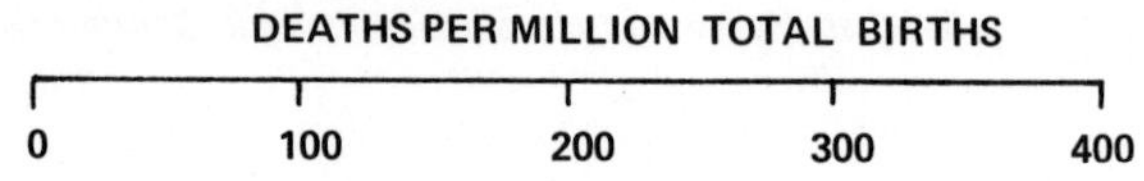

FIG. 1. Maternal deaths by social class (all deaths between 1965 and 1971). Scotland: deaths per million total births.

Some evidence is also displayed in relation to morbidity and disability.

These social class differences are not limited to mortality and morbidity. They run through the gamut of physical attributes upon which estimates are made of normal healthy development—for example there are differences in birth weights and persisting differences in height and weight in school children.

Much discussion turns on the question of whether these well known social class differences are or are not diminishing. For the most part the evidence suggests that the gaps remain as wide apart as a generation ago and in some instances the gaps may be widening. This persistence of

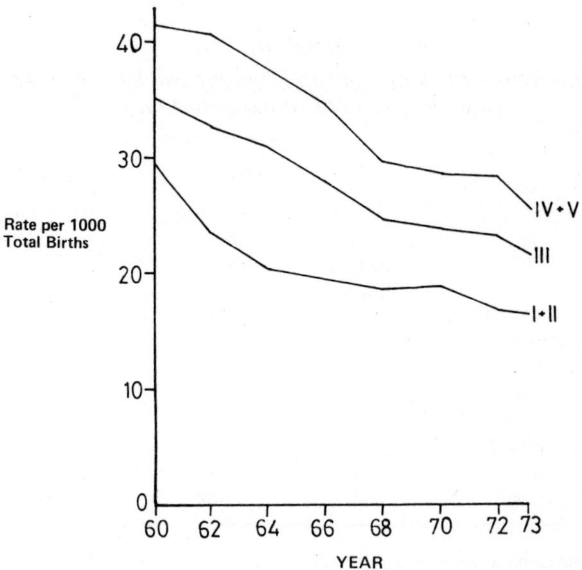

FIG. 2. Legitimate perinatal mortality per 1,000 total births by social class. Scotland 1960–73. From Scottish Registrar General's Data.

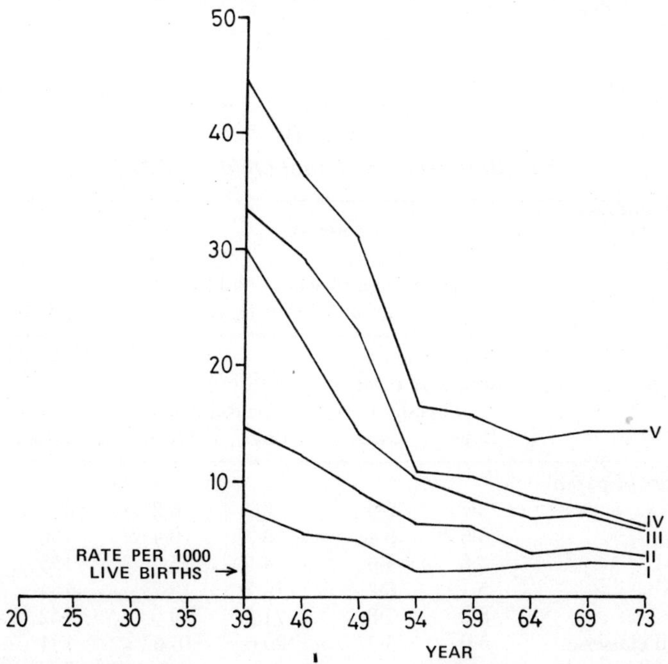

FIG. 3. Post-neonatal deaths per 1,000 live births by social class Scotland. From Scottish Registrar General's Data.

TABLE III

Males reporting illness by social group England and Wales 1972. Observed rates as per cent of expected rates

	Chronic sickness		Acute sickness
	Long-standing illness	Limiting long-standing illness	Restricted activity in a two-week period
Professional	87	74	87
Employers	84	78	91
Intermediate	92	86	93
Skilled manual	103	103	101
Semi-skilled	117	120	111
Unskilled	136	156	151
All groups	100	100	100

From Central Statistical Office (1975).
Source: General Household Survey Annual Report 1972.

TABLE IV

Health defects in school children, 1973

	Scotland					
	Percentages of school children at the age of 5 suffering from				Height of school children at the age of 14 (cm)	
	Uncorrected refractive error in eyesight		Dental care			
	Boys	Girls	Boys	Girls	Boys	Girls
Social class of parent						
I	3·7	2·9	6·7	8·2	158	156
II	3·6	5·4	8·3	9·4	156	156
III	4·6	4·6	14·5	15·7	155	155
IV	5·1	6·2	16·7	19·7	154	154
V	8·6	7·8	21·2	20·6	152	153
All classes	5·0	5·3	20·6	16·6	154	154

Source: Scottish Information Services Division.

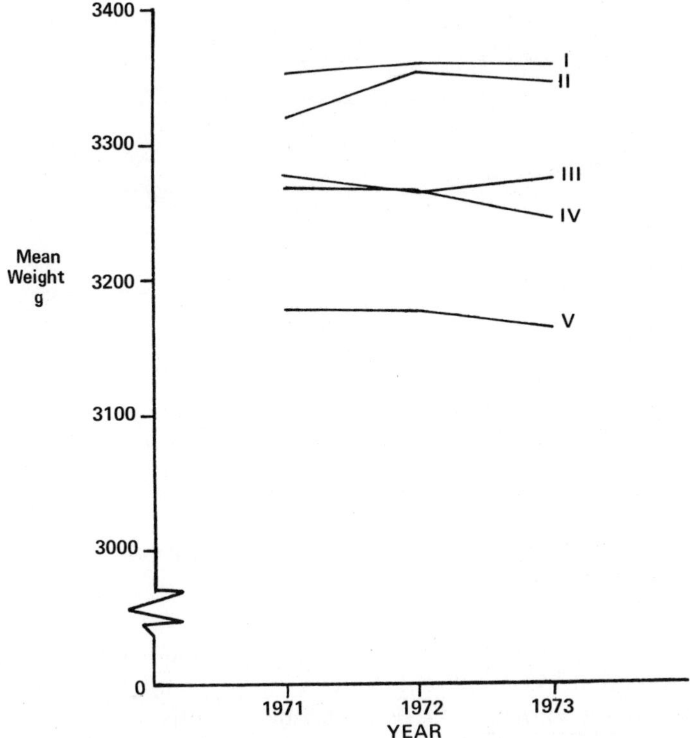

FIG. 4. Mean birth weight and social class. Scotland 1971–73. Source: Scottish Information Services Division.

difference and the possibility that in some instances differences may be growing greater has been a source of perplexity and disappointment to those who believe in the National Health Service as a means of bringing improved health and more equal opportunities for health within our communities (Butler and Bonham, 1963).

What do these differences mean? Do they mean that the National Health Service has totally failed in a main purpose during its generation or more of life? I will hope to demonstrate later that this is much too sweeping a conclusion to draw but these social class differences must remain in front of us all and the Health Service planner in particular as a challenge to study the reasons and to draw the appropriate conclusions and responses from them.

It is to be noticed that there are other indices of unequal experience in health as well as the social class differences which are of great impor-

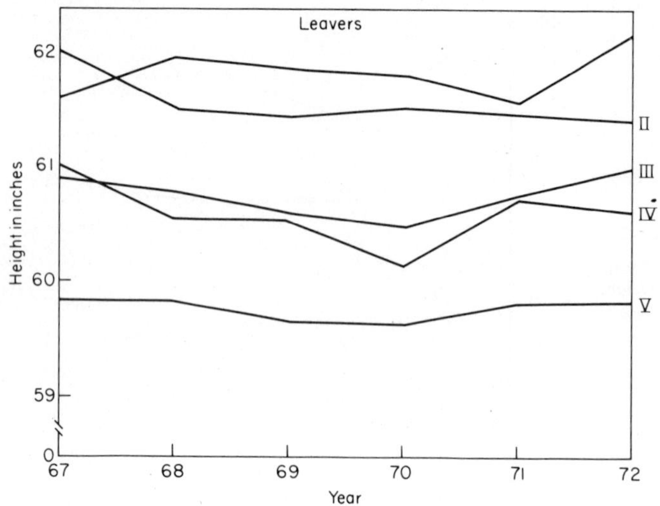

FIG. 5. Heights of school leavers (boys) in social class. Scotland 1967–72. Source: Scottish Information Services Division.

tance in our thinking for the future. For example—the differences in health experience in different regions of the country—these are also now becoming known—*Which* magazine recently discussed and displayed them in an article about the health service (1975). From my point of view the most notable difference is the more generally adverse health experience in Scotland as compared with other parts of the United Kingdom and especially the more prosperous South of England; but there are similar differences within Scotland and between the regions within England. Within the regions the social class differences exist and persist as for the country as a whole but there are also marked differences in experience between social classes in different regions (Illsley, 1967; Illsley and Kincard, 1963). For example, in the regions with the more adverse experience the health experience of social class I corresponds approximately to the health experience of social class III in the regions with better health indices. This evidence must equally be a challenge to the health planner and I will discuss it briefly later.

Use of Services

To what extent is there evidence of inequality or at any rate difference in use of services by different social groups? There has been a good deal of discussion about this since the early days of the National Health Service

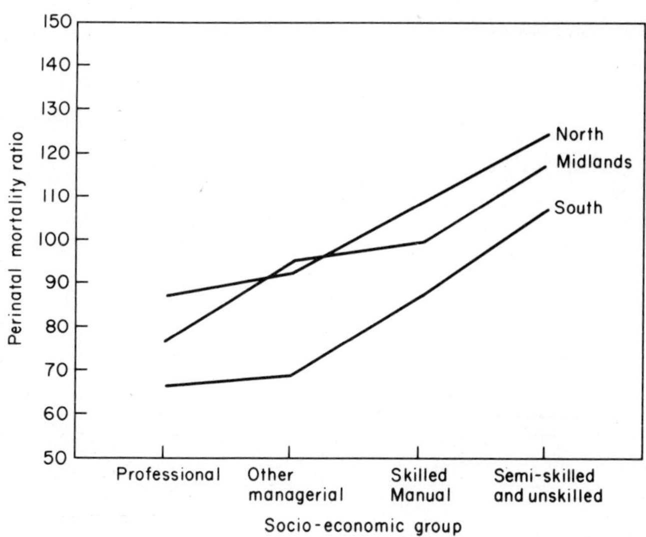

FIG. 6. Perinatal death rates in each region and socio-economic group in Great Britain in 1958 expressed as a ratio of the national rate (Great Britain = 100).
From Illsley (1967).
Source: British Perinatal Mortality Survey 1958.

TABLE V

Death rates per 1,000 population at ages 35–64 in England and Wales and Scotland by social class. Males 1959–63.

		35–44	45–54	55–64
Social class I	England and Wales	1·7	5·4	17·0
	Scotland	2·1	7·6	21·1
Social class II	England and Wales	1·8	5·5	18·2
	Scotland	2·5	7·8	21·9
Social class III	England and Wales	2·3	7·1	22·2
	Scotland	2·7	8·4	25·1
Social class IV	England and Wales	2·5	7·3	22·0
	Scotland	3·2	8·9	24·8
Social class V	England and Wales	4·4	11·2	29·1
	Scotland	5·9	13·4	34·1

From Heasman (unpublished paper).

TABLE VI

Infant mortality rates per 1,000 live births by social class for Scottish cities: 1961 and 1970

	Aberdeen		Glasgow	
Social class	1961	1970	1961	1970
I and II	18·4	10·0	24·5	15·8
III	19·2	14·6	28·8	18·2
IV and V	29·9	16·0	34·7	32·9
IV and V as a percentage of I and II	163·0	160·0	142·0	248·0

Source: Registrar General for Scotland.

when Titmuss drew attention to differences in use of services and drew the conclusion that middle class members of the community were more efficient in the use of the National Health Service and were getting greater benefits from it (Titmuss, 1969). Some of the differences of view in discussion may perhaps stem from a tendency to draw conclusions about total use of the health services from evidence in relation to one particular service. Recently McKinlay has drawn our attention to the fact that there may be different patterns of behaviour in relation to different services (McKinlay, 1970). In other words we should not draw conclusions about total health service use from evidence in relation to one particular service.

The evidence suggests on the whole that the amount of use and effectiveness of use of the different parts of the health service varies with social class and generally speaking in the direction of less use being made as we go down in the social scale. This is however by no means clear in relation to the use of hospital beds in Scotland. There has been clear demonstration that our general acute hospital beds are used more by the lower social groups; not only in terms of numbers of admissions but even more so in terms of total bed days (Carstairs and Patterson, 1966). This does not necessarily mean that the groups concerned make an amount of use which corresponds to their greater morbidity experience. We do not have the kinds of evidence of need which enable us to come to a conclusion on this point but Vera Carstairs in discussing this evidence suggested that some at least of the difference in bed usage might arise from a need to compensate for poorer housing and greater domestic difficulties as well as for greater morbidity. When we look at consultations with the general practitioner we do not have much direct evidence in Scotland and I have gone to other sources; for example the

TABLE VII

Hospital standardized discharge ratios in Scotland: 1963

Males	SDR	Females	SDR
Class I	92·5	Class I	98·6
II	84·1	II	95·0
III	91·7	III	92·0
IV	105·4	IV	100·0
V	148·8	V	155·5
ALL	100·0	ALL	100·0

The standardized discharge ratio is based on a measure for each class of what the rate would be if the age structure for each class was the same as in the classified population generally; this figure is then expressed as a percentage of the rates in the population generally.

The data covers all Scottish hospitals except maternity, mental and mental deficiency hospitals.
From Carstairs and Patterson (1966).
Source: Scottish Hospital In-Patient Statistics.

TABLE VIII

Hospital standardized mean stay ratios in Scotland: 1963

Males	SMSR	Females	SMSR
Class I	77·5	Class I	88·2
II	88·2	II	93·3
III	98·7	III	99·4
IV	103·0	IV	102·8
V	112·1	V	106·8
ALL	100·0	ALL	100·0

SMRS = Standarized mean stay ratio which is based on mean stay in days is calculated in the same way as the standardized discharge ratio.

The data covers all Scottish hospitals except maternity, mental and mental deficiency.
From Carstairs and Patterson (1966)
Source: Scottish Hospital In-Patient Statistics.

General Household Survey, evidence from Ann Cartwright's survey studies and the morbidity recording study of Logan and Cushion. Here the evidence shows for the adult male an increase in frequency of consultations with the general practitioner as we go down the scale of social classes. This picture is particularly clear at working ages. It tends to change in the other direction after retirement. This picture is not so clear-cut for females. This is bound to raise the question in our minds as to what extent this gradient is determined by requirements for certification for sickness benefit rather than by the simple equation of general practice to the morbidity needs of the situation. Nor is it clear that the greater frequency of use of the general practitioner as we move down the social scale effectively corresponds to the needs of social groups with greater morbidity experience. Attempts have been made to create a crude ratio of service to need by relating frequency of consultation to indices of sickness; such attempts tend to demonstrate that the more

TABLE IX

Use of health services—persons consulting a GP (NHS) in a two-week period by social group 1972. Scotland, England and Wales

	Males		Females	
	Scotland	England and Wales	Scotland	England and Wales
Professional and employers	91·4	93·5	144·3	111·6
Intermediate and junior N/M	109·2	90·5	127·1	133·7
Skilled manual	121·9	94·6	141·8	132·5
Semi and unskilled manual	112·5	121·4	141·9	133·7

Source: General Household Survey 1972.

TABLE X

Use/need ratio by social group

Scotland and England and Wales 1972

Social Group	Scotland	England and Wales
Professionals	100	133
Employers/managers	109	92
Intermediate and junior N/M	87	77
Skilled manual	57	63
Semi-skilled manual	66	71
Unskilled	34	57

From data in General Household Survey tables for Scotland and England and Wales 1972.
* i.e. the ratio of the number of general practioner consultations to the number of restricted activity days (both sexes) in two weeks.

TABLE XI

General practioner consultation rates per 1,000 population by social class and age

	Children under 15 by fathers' occupation per 1,000 pop.	Men aged 15–64 Consultation rates per 1,000 pop.
Social class	Consultations	Consultations
1	2,832	2,165
2	2,958	2,506
3	3,231	3,091
4	3,063	3,431
5	2.972	3,701
TOTAL	3,109	3,069

Quoted by Rein (1969).
Source: Logan (1960).

TABLE XII

Children less than 5 by social group. England and Wales 1972.

Rate per 1,000 consulting a G.P. (NHS) in a 2-week period

SOCIAL GROUP	MALE	FEMALE
Professional/employers	141·1	152·5
Intermediate and junior N.M.	123·0	152·7
Skilled manual	124·1	158·5
Semi and unskilled manual	159·9	125·0

Average number of consultations per person per year

SOCIAL GROUP	MALE	FEMALE
Professional/employers	4·2	4·9
Intermediate and junior N.M.	3·7	4·7
Skilled manual	4·5	5·3
Semi and unskilled manual	4·5	3·5

Source: General Household Survey 1972.

frequent consultations reported does not match the greater level of morbidity experience in lower social groups.

When we look at the evidence on the frequency of consultation with the general practitioner for children there is little difference in the reported frequency of use by the social groups (Office of Population Censuses and Surveys, 1975). This is an item of evidence which must raise some anxiety. We know the evidence of increased mortality and morbidity in children in lower social groups. Furthermore, we know that of deaths occurring among young children in social class V a considerable proportion occur at home (Douglas 1971; Richards, 1971). For children the evidence suggests that there may be factors preventing the most effective use of general practitioner services by the lowest social groups.

I will not discuss to any extent dental health and use of dental services but there is much evidence to demonstrate the serious fall in levels of dental health in the United Kingdom as we move down the social scale and equally evidence to show the less effective use of dental services in the same direction.

In discussing what one might call the purely clinical services the evidence on use by social class is not all in one direction. When we move to consider what might be called the clinical promotive services the picture is more clear-cut. These services, for example the maternity and child welfare services, involve a more considerable element of individual decision and initiative than do the purely disease related services. In the disease related services, particularly those for acute illness—the individual is perhaps more driven by his or her signs and symptoms in the direction of the service, whereas with the clinical promotive services he or she or the family are more involved in determining not only whether to use the service but when to use it.

The maternity service makes an interesting study in its own right in such matters and I will refer again to this later in relation to Aberdeen. In general we can note that the statistics of use of the maternity service by social class have improved over the years as more services have become available. As we move towards a 100 per cent hospitalization for childbirth we move away from the situation of the recent past where it was often true that those groups in greatest need of hospitalization were least likely to get it whether from their own decision or because of service deployments. But even now contact with the maternity services varies with social groups. Those social groups in greatest need are least likely to come early to the notice of the service for antenatal care. There may also be hospital delays in seeing the antenatal patient and although these are not necessarily greater for lower social groups they will bear hardest on those who tend to come latest for care (McIllwaine, 1974).

In relation to use of child welfare services the evidence is much in the same direction (Davie, *et al.*, 1972; Richards, 1971). Lower social groups make less use of the child welfare clinics and those who need them most,

TABLE XIII
Late ante-natal booking.
Per cent of married women in each social class making an ante-natal booking more than 20 weeks of gestation (excluding women whose date of last menstrual period is uncertain)

Scotland 1971–73

	1971	1972	1973
I	28·4	27·2	27·0
II	35·3	32·3	29·8
III	36·3	33·4	30·6
IV	39·3	37·8	35·3
V	47·1	44·2	40·5

Source: Scottish Information Services Division.

for example the mothers with larger families, are least likely to make use of them. There is evidence that the health services which are perhaps most specifically geared to the purpose of health promotion amongst groups in greatest need do not always succeed in deploying themselves appropriately for this purpose. Nor do health visiting services necessarily fully compensate (Cartwright and O'Brien, 1976). We rightly look to the health visitor as the most important member of the health team in reaching out to those with greatest need. Yet there is no clear evidence of positive discrimination in the deployment of the health visitor's time in the direction of groups in greatest need.

The evidence in relation to preventive services, for example for immunization, goes in the same direction (Gordon, 1951). The take-up of immunization against specific diseases and indeed other kinds of take-ups such as welfare foods suggests that it is the more privileged social groups who make most use of the services available. This is a particularly instructive example of the differences in social class behaviour in relation to the health services. Here are services where on the whole initiative has been needed by the individual parent in making use of the service. It is apparently those with clearest information about the relation of the service to health and with the clearest concept of the effect of actions today in relation to benefits in the future who make most use of the service. Changes in deployment of services which diminish the need for individual initiative (for example computer controlled immunization programmes) diminish the difference in take-ups between social groups. There are instructive lessons to be drawn from this.

TABLE XIV

Use of health services by children < 7 by social class (of father)—Great Britain 1965

	I	II	IIIN	IIIM	IV	V
Per cent who had never visited a dentist	16	20	19	24	27	31
Per cent not immunized against:						
Smallpox	6	14	16	25	29	33
Polio	1	3	3	4	6	10
Diphtheria	1	3	3	6	8	11

Source: The Second Report of the National Child Development Study (1958, Cohort).

Use of Maternity Services in Aberdeen

Before moving to discuss in more detail the reasons for differences in social class morbidity experience and behaviour in relation to health services and what might be done about this, I believe it will be instructive to pause and look at some of the experience from maternity services in Aberdeen.

I base my discussion on the assumption with which I hope you will agree that the Aberdeen maternity service as structured by Sir Dugald Baird can be taken as an example (perhaps the best example anywhere) of a well planned, well led, socially orientated health service. Dugald Baird has discussed in a number of papers the elements of a well planned maternity service which should integrate into one team policy all the essential hospital and community elements of the service and whose efforts should be planned on sound epidemiological evidence of the best ways and times and places of deploying service in relation to needs (Baird, 1969).

The results of Dugald Baird's policies in Aberdeen are well known. Despite a situation in which the environmental and social characteristics of the population served were by no means ideal (for example the social class distribution and the physique of the mothers was considerably less advantageous to health service results than those in the South of England) results have been achieved in terms of measurable indices such as perinatal mortality rates which compare with the best in the United Kingdom (Baird, 1973). It has also been demonstrated in the city of Dundee that when the same principles and practices were taken elsewhere into a community with a good deal of adverse circumstances similar results were soon achieved.

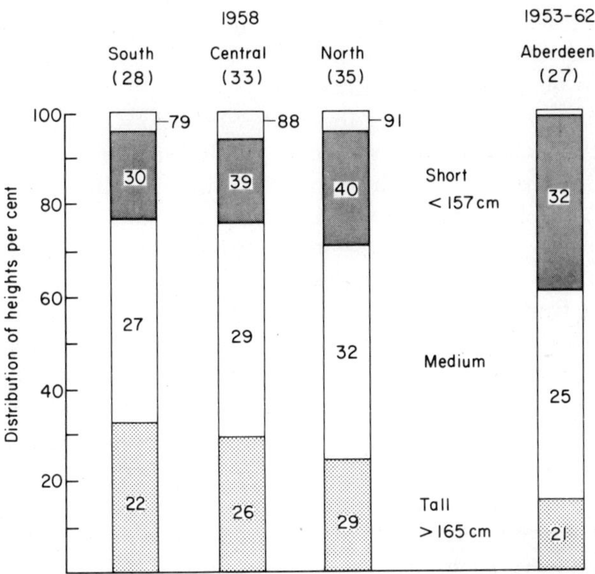

FIG. 7. Perinatal mortality survey. Source: Baird (1973).

TABLE XV

Perinatal mortality rates per 1,000 total births for Scottish cities, 1950, 1960 and 1970

	1950		1960		1970	
	Perinatal mortality rate	Per cent of Aberdeen	Perinatal mortality rate	Per cent of Aberdeen	Perinatal mortality rate	Per cent of Aberdeen
Aberdeen	37	100	32	100	20	100
Dundee	52	141	32	100	19	95
Edinburgh	39	105	33	103	22	110
Glasgow	48	130	42	131	28	140

Source: Registrar General for Scotland. Scottish Information Services Division.

At the start of these policies in Aberdeen the familiar social gradient in experience for example in perinatal death rates was evident. What was the situation when Sir Dugald retired? What is the situation today after a generation or more of this highly developed policy of deployment of service in relation to need? The overall situation is much improved, all social groups have benefited. But the social class gradient in perinatal death rates is as wide as ever (Baird, 1974b). What are the messages to be drawn from this fact?

In examining this evidence from Aberdeen do we draw some kind of pessimistic conclusion that whatever our efforts may be we still find ourselves standing in the same place? I do not think so at all. The message I take from the Aberdeen experience and I believe it to be a most important message is this—to a considerable extent our impact in relation to the lower social classes and their more adverse experience has to come from a total effort in each area and region whereby we plan more effectively to allocate and deploy our resources to the needs of the situations. In such circumstances it is true that benefits will come to all social groups and will not be specifically received only by the least privileged. The gap in experience between the most privileged and the least privileged will persist but what is of great importance is that the total experience of each social group will be improved.

Let us remember also at this point the evidence showing the difference in health experience in different regions and the differences in health experience between the same social classes in different regions. In other words the opportunity for advance by improved deployment of resources ranges across all social groups in regions with more adverse health experience.

The most important step is to achieve more equal deployments of resources and efforts between the different parts of the country. What we very much need is better indices of need on which to base this redeployment. Do not imagine that in any way I underestimate the difficulties of achieving this redeployment especially at a time of very limited economic growth in the health service. But we must be clear what we have to do—even if it is difficult and will take time.

Why does the Social Class Gap Persist?

I do not suppose anybody imagines that I can advance a solution to this question which has occupied the minds of much better qualified social analysts than I am, but it may be useful to attempt a review of some of the possible elements of an answer to see if they can give us guidance in relation to action for the future.

DEFINITIONS OF SOCIAL CLASS

I have been much instructed by the analyses and writings in a number of papers of Raymond Illsley on this subject (Illsley, 1955; 1967). You will remember that he analysed in relation to the experience of mothers in Aberdeen the movement on marriage between social classes. He demonstrated an upward social trend of women who were taller and healthier and opposite movement of less healthy and smaller females. He also demonstrated that the women who moved up the social scale in this way had less perinatal mortality than those who moved down. In fact the demonstration was of a process of selective mating leading to reinforcement of upper social groups with healthier recruits and with opposite effects at the lowest end of the social scale. Here is a kind of homoeostatic mechanism which affects the evidence on health experience presented when we analyse by the Registrar General's social groups. On this basis the groups are so defined as to be kept continuously apart in their health experience so long as we have social mobility in our communities.

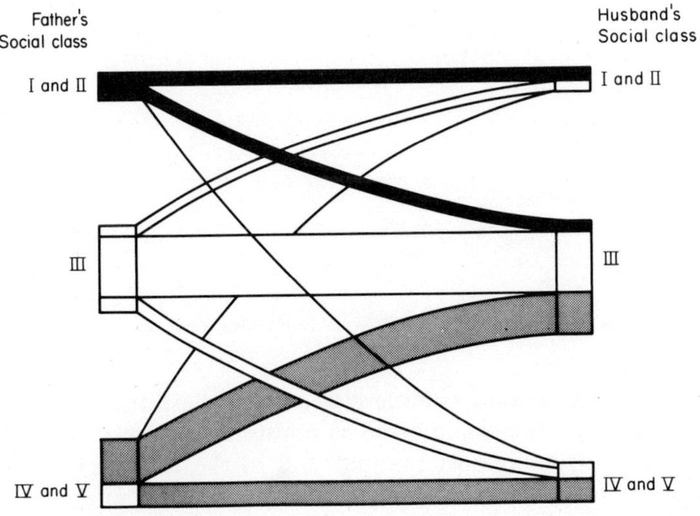

Fig. 8. Intermarriage between social classes. Aberdeen married primiparae, 1950–54. The breadth of the lines is proportional to the numbers in each group.
From Illsley (1955).

What is the message to be drawn from this analysis? One point to make is that Registrar General's data on social class difference cannot be used as a datum point against which to measure the impact over time of the National Health Service and other services on the health of differential social groups in our community. We know that in our

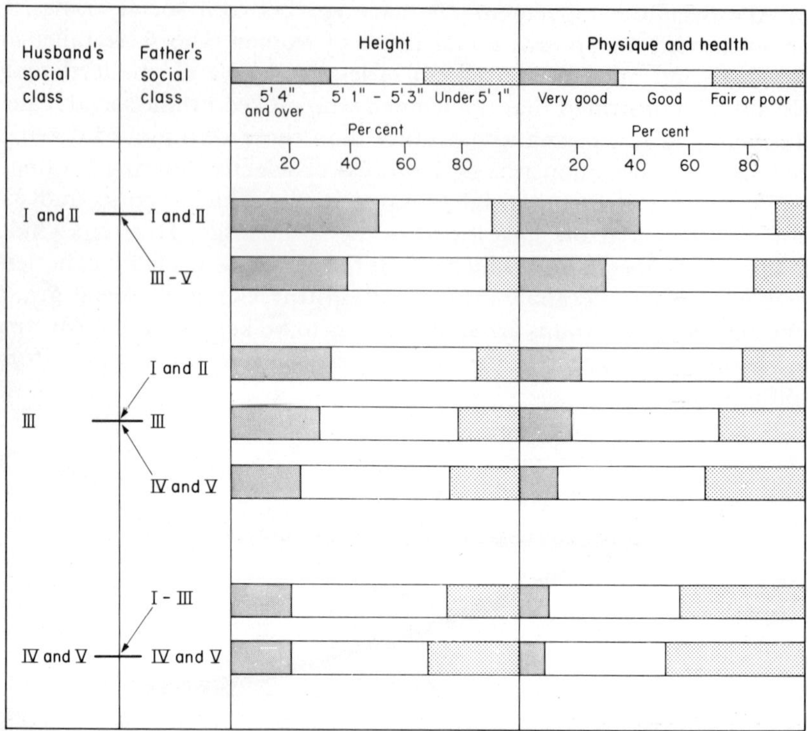

FIG. 9. Inter-class movement—height, physique and health. From Illsley (1955).

changing industrial and commercial society there has been a steady increase in the numbers employed in non-manual occupations (including professional) as against manual and in the numbers occupied in skilled as opposed to unskilled work. These increased numbers in what are recorded as higher social groups have been recruited from individuals whose origins lay in lower social groups. Looking at the community as a whole and most of its social elements it is certain that health experience has improved and that the various elements of our National Health Service have played a part in this. But if we wish a fixed point against which to measure exactly progress in terms of National Health Service impacts on socially influenced health problems we will have to find this elsewhere than by the traditional analysis of social class difference.

On the other hand, I draw the conclusion that for the health planner

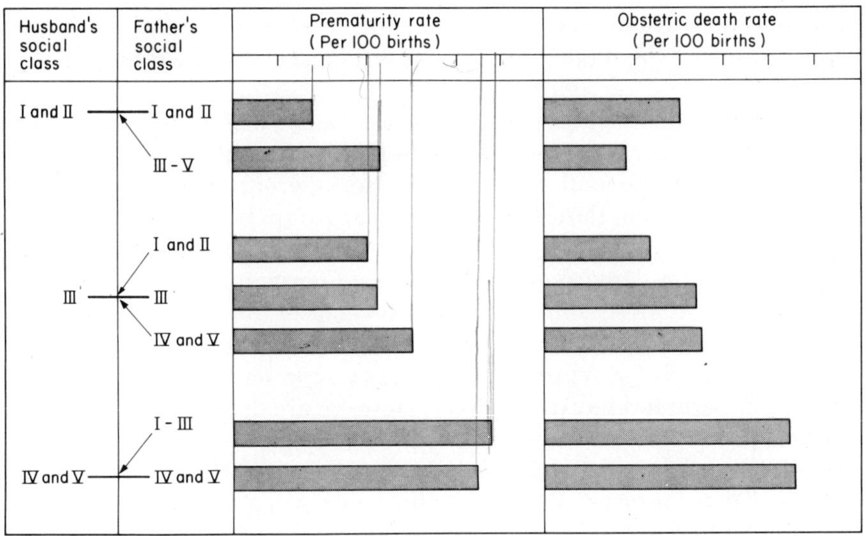

FIG. 10. Inter-class movement—premature and obstetric death rate. From Illsley (1955).

the traditional social class analysis remains as instructive as ever—perhaps more so. The dynamic processes of social mobility have the effect of concentrating at the lowest end of the social scale groups which are recruited and reinforced in a fashion which makes them most subject to morbidity and least able and least likely to make use of available resources to help themselves. It is as if we were having identified for us those for whom the traditional assumptions of the National Health Service are least effective. I take the message that these analyses are a challenge to us to find ways and means of deploying some of our efforts differently, and specifically to bring the services to groups who cannot or will not use them to best advantage themselves.

BIOLOGICAL EFFECTS OF DEPRIVATION

The biological effects of deprivation on physical constitution and health are not limited to reproductive efficiency but they are perhaps best recorded in that field. The demonstrations by Baird and his colleagues of differential reproductive efficiency in relation to maternal height and physique are well known. They have also divided perinatal deaths (which of course includes stillbirths) by cause into two main groups.

"Obstetric"* where the deaths are primarily affected by the effectiveness of obstetric care and "environmental"† where the causes lie in the constitution of the mother and all the circumstances which have determined this.

The fall in death rates due to obstetric causes has been greater than for the environmental group. Even in relation to "obstetric" causes of perinatal death the mothers from upper social groups may benefit more from good care than those from lower social groups because their general physique is better.

In relation to "environmental" causes of perinatal death the picture is different and more complex. The social class gradient is wider and the opportunities within present knowledge for improvements are much more restricted. "Environmental" causes represent two-thirds of the factors in perinatal mortality today. Here we are dealing with causes of perinatal mortality and morbidity which lie in the constitutional make-up of the mothers involving all the factors which have led to their physical development. We are dealing with circumstances where the effects of difference in social backgrounds and experience go back a long time and are much more ingrained and slow to change (Baird, 1975b). It is noteworthy that Baird has now turned his attention to evidence which suggests that recent increases in perinatal death rates in certain social groups in Aberdeen and elsewhere from "environmental" causes (showing themselves for example in congenital malformation deaths and deaths associated with low birth weight) could perhaps be tied back to the early upbringing of the mothers during periods of economic depression. He suggests that social deprivations in early life have an impact on constitution and reproductive efficiency which demonstrates itself much later when the women come to childbirth. Baird has further suggested on his evidence that the female children of women born in these circumstances may themselves have a lesser reproductive efficiency as demonstrated in terms of higher perinatal death rates from environmental causes. He speculates that this could be due to constitutional damage carrying itself into a second generation or it could be due to patterns of behaviour which are passed from mother to daugher (Baird, 1973: 1974a; 1974b).

* The Obstetric group consists of deaths from pre-eclampsia, mechanical complications of labour, "unexplained" deaths of babies weighing over 2,500 gm, deaths due to ante-partum haemorrhage, and those due to Rhesus incompatability.

† The environmental groups consists of "unexplained" deaths of babies weighing less than 2,500 gm, deaths from congenital malformations, and those related primarily to diseases in the mother.

There is some overlap between the groups since the devitalized baby of the less robust mother is less able to withstand hazards of obstetric complications.

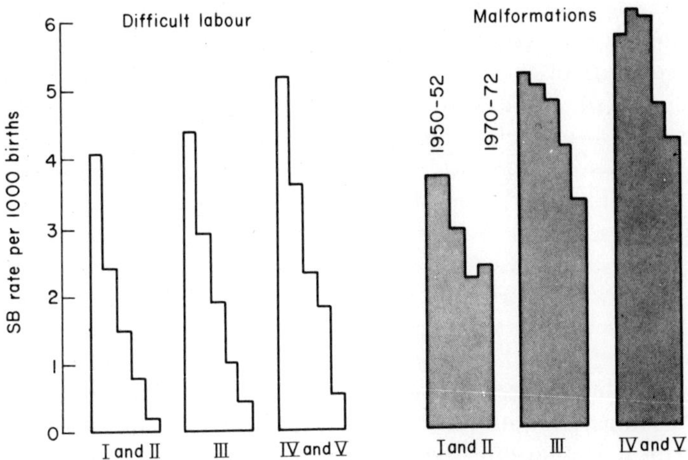

FIG. 11. Stillbirth rate: difficult labour and malformations. Scotland in 1950–52, 53–57, 60–62, 65–67, 70–72. From Baird (1975b).

TABLE XVI

Perinatal mortality rate, para O, environmental and obstetric causes by social class, in 5-year groups 1948–72

	Environmental				Obstetric			
Years	I–IIIa	IIIb,c	IV+V	All	I–IIIa	IIIb,c	IV+V	All
1946–47	—	—	—	22·5	—	—	—	32·3
1948–52	16·1	16·1	31·3	21·7	22·0	17·8	18·9	20·4
1953–57	9·6	18·2	16·3	13·7	14·7	15·4	22·5	16·8
1958–62	17·1	13·9	15·3	15·8	11·7	15·6	12·3	13·8
1963–67	16·1	16·3	17·1	15·1	8·5	12·2	12·3	13·0
1968–72	7·9	12·4	29·8	15·6	5·1	6·3	12·6	7·6
per cent fall 1948–52 to 1968–72	51·0	23·0	5·0	28·0	77·0	65·0	33·0	63·0

From Baird (1974b).

INFLUENCE OF INTELLIGENCE AND EDUCATION

It would be surprising if intelligence and education are not helpful in making better and more effective use of the various elements of the National Health Service and we might expect to find this most clearly demonstrated in those parts of the service which, because of their preventive and promotive nature, are presented least urgently as far as the individual is concerned. Ann Cartwright with O'Brien has recently reviewed some of the evidence from her own studies (Cartwright and O'Brien, 1976). For example—where individuals were asked a number of questions about different diseases the proportion of right answers to questions was considerably higher in social class I respondents than those in social class V. Similar evidence was demonstrated in relation to knowledge about birth control methods. Individuals from professional social groups were more critical of health services and more prepared to voice their criticism about these health services, and one might presume were also more prepared to intervene to try to have the service improved as far as they themselves were concerned. The professional class respondents were also more likely than those of lower social groups to ask pertinent questions in relation to their own condition.

We can note that effective co-operation and response in relation to a number of important issues of preventive medicine and curative regimes today requires intelligent, informed and sustained co-operation by the individual. This is certainly true in relation to the modern plagues which can be attributed to smoking, alcohol and overeating. It is also true in relation to the pursuit of almost any regime to control a chronic disorder, for example the care of diabetes. It will be even more true if and when we move on any scale into screening programmes for early detection of disease.

I use the term "fashion trend" to illustrate the way in which public behaviour will move in relation to health needs. It is probable that as with other fashion trends new practices will move from the upper social classes downwards. This has been well demonstrated in relation to family planning. The importance of family planning in improving the maternity and infant health experience of lower social groups cannot be over-emphasized. Family planning started with the upper social groups and has moved rather slowly (but with increasing acceleration) to those who need it most. Evidence in relation to smoking points in the same direction. Self reported behaviour in relation to smoking today shows that it is to an increasing extent a lower class habit and to a diminishing extent practised by more privileged groups. Perhaps the most ironical example of the effects of fashion is to be found in relation to programmes for screening for carcinoma of the cervix where just those groups (i.e. women from upper social classes) who are least likely to develop cancer of the cervix are also most likely to present themselves for screening. Incidentally, the Aberdeen programme of MacGregor is a good example of how one has to respond to this kind of situation by

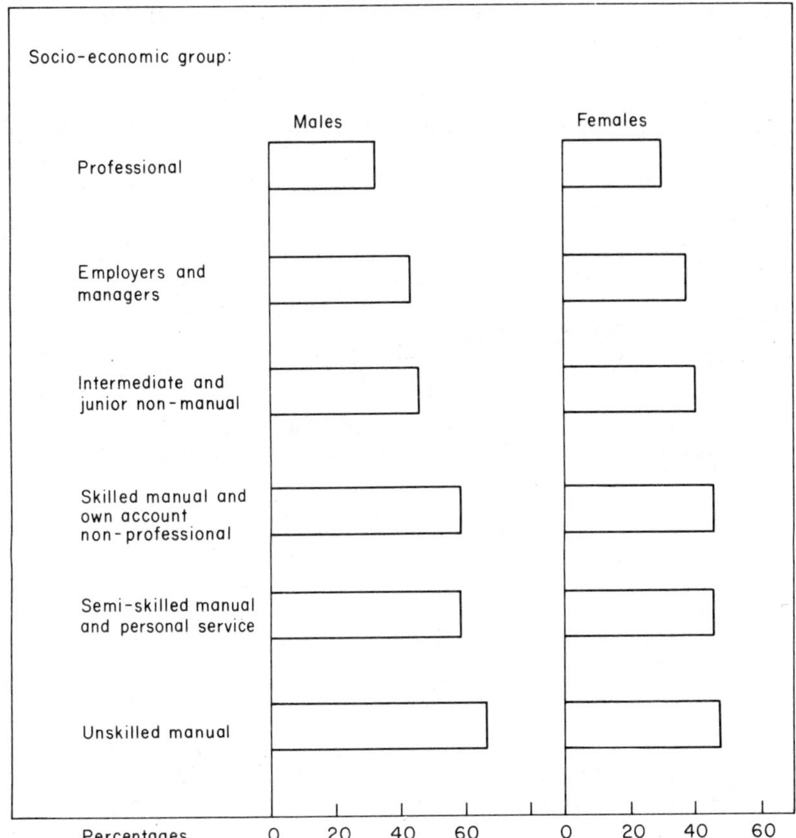

Fig. 12. Current cigarette smokers by socio-economic group, 1973. (Standardized for age.) Source: General Household Survey. Classification: GHS socio-economic groupings of own occupation except for married women where it is husband's occupation.

developing methods of deployment which take the service to those in greatest need (MacGregor and Baird, 1963). It should perhaps be noted that the effects of fashion are not always to the advantage of those who pioneer. Glover demonstrated in the 1920s that at that time tribal custom dictated a virtually 100 per cent tonsillectomy in upper social groups. It was only those in the lowest social groups who had any chance of preserving their tonsils into adult life. We are now very much more sceptical about the value of tonsillectomy and today it seems to be a fashion progressively abandoned by upper social groups and to a greater proportional extent practised among lower social class children.

BEHAVIOUR AND VALUE SYSTEMS

This is an umbrella heading under which I discuss a number of complicated factors. At the back of differences in use of health services must lie important differences in the value systems of the groups concerned. These in turn derive from the culture in which they were brought up. They determine behaviour particularly in relation to the use of services which relate to such matters as child bearing and child rearing. McKinlay has depicted these in diagrammatic form (McKinlay, 1970).

TABLE XVII

Utilization of maternity and child welfare service. Diagrammatic representation of a conceptual framework.

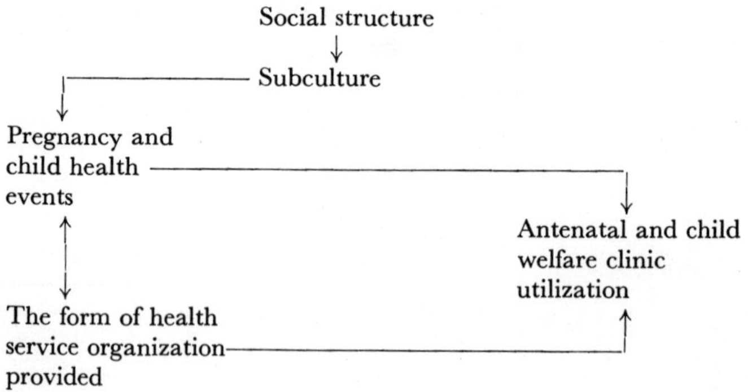

There are traditional patterns of behaviour which persist even when apparently harmful to the individual or her offspring. For example—the reluctance of the working class mother with several children to come into hospital for confinement and her preference for domiciliary confinement. No doubt she has her own reasons for this preference but in purely obstetric terms domiciliary confinement for her is dangerous. Family size alone is bound to be a major factor in determining the ability of a mother to make use of infant welfare services so long as use of them depends solely on her initiative and her ability to take her child to a clinic.

Illsley has commented on the effects of time lag (Illsley, 1967; Illsley and Kincaid, 1963). He notes that you may change methods of treatment and availability of health services and even income without necessarily getting appropriate response to these changes quickly. There are factors in the environment such as housing and urban conditions generally. There are personal matters such as habits of hygiene, methods of infant care and the whole attitude to health facilities which do not necessarily change rapidly. Indeed Illsley suggests in the short run it may be the educated middle class who will benefit most from new developments and opportunities because their education enables them to take immediate advantage of improved medical and social services. If this is so we may get decreasing total death or morbidity rates initially accompanied by widened class differentials and only later a gradual tendency towards equalization.

Another element in this complex matter is the difference in behaviour to be found within social classes which the conventional Registrar General social class definitions will not tell us about. For example in Newcastle within the large manual class III as wide differences in health and use of health services could be found between families defined by the health visitors as efficient and families defined as inefficient as could be found in the whole range of social class experience between the extremes of class I and class V (Nelignan *et al.*, 1974). McKinlay in a detailed study of a small number of social class V utilizers and underutilizers of maternity services identified difference in the whole life style of the two groups. (McKinlay and McKinlay, 1972.) The utilizers on the whole planned their lives, the underutilizers were identified as crisis motivated.

HEALTH SERVICE DEPLOYMENTS

There are clearly elements determining differences in health service usage which are related to the deployments of the health service itself and the attitudes of health workers.

There are questions of access as far as health promotive services are concerned and it may be much more difficult for mothers in low income groups to mobilize the time and effort to make use of these services so long as access depends solely on their initiative.

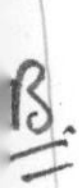

More broadly speaking the health service in its major deployment and underlying philosophy is a self-help service. It operates on the assumption that if the services are made available individuals in need will use them. No doubt for the most part this is a correct assumption. But equally if our most severe and reactionary health problems are found in social groups for whom these assumptions are not warranted we must be prepared to re-examine the assumptions and draw appropriate conclusions in relation to the groups and services for whom the "self-help" system does not operate effectively. We require policies of positive discrimination in the direction of greatest need. And since such positive discrimination runs counter to the normal flow of our efforts, it is essential to monitor to ensure that the desired deployment in fact takes place.

Recently Douglas after discussing comparisons in relation to maternal and infant child health between the findings of his own survey in 1946 and the similar evidence from the Birthday Trust Survey of 1958, drew the conclusion that on a number of important matters affecting deprived groups there seemed to have been little progress during that period of 12 years despite improvement in the population as a whole (Douglas, 1971). Indeed he suggested that in some respect things might have deteriorated for the deprived groups. From this he drew the conclusion that it is insufficient simply to provide better services or to assume that they will be fully used by those who most require them; we have also to make sure that these services are appropriately deployed and are really used by those in greatest need. If other sections of the community already better provided take the services over and make use of them then the group for which they were specially intended will suffer a relative deterioration in the level of care received.

There are elements in usage of health services which may be affected by the social rapport between health professionals and their patients. For the most part health professionals come from middle class backgrounds. It would be somewhat surprising in these circumstances if they did not make easier rapport with middle class patients. Unless the health professionals are aware of this possibility bias may emerge. Ann Cartwright has commented on this. In her studies she found that general practitioners knew more about their middle class patients. The middle class patient is more likely to regard his doctor as a peer and to be more confident of the importance of his own problems in dealing with his doctor. So far as difference in service provision was concerned domiciliary visits arranged by the general practitioner for elderly patients in terminal illness were more frequently arranged for middle class patients than for lower class patients. Also the general practitioner was more likely to visit his middle class patients in hospital. The proportion of direct admissions to hospital was 45 per cent for general practitioners middle class patients and 35 per cent amongst working class patients (Cartwright and O'Brien, 1976). Buchan and Richardson in Aberdeen also showed that there was a social class gradient in the duration of the consultation time of general practitioners with their patients with somewhat longer periods spent with upper social class patients (Buchan and Richardson, 1971).

Important elements of the health service in deprived environments may be less well provided than those available in better-off communities. There are clear difficulties for the patient or the parent in circumstances where lock-up general practice surgeries predominate. Communication after hours has to be by telephone call sometimes with a necessity to work through referred phone numbers in surroundings where public telephones may be vandalized. The difficulties are not diminished for individuals whose education and experience in handling complicated situations is limited. Information under this heading is not well documented but again there is some evidence from Ann Cartwright's studies of general practitioners (Cartwright, 1964; Cartwright and Marshall, 1965). She found that in predominately working areas 80 per cent of the doctors surgeries were built before 1900 whereas in middle class areas fewer than 50 per cent of the surgeries have been built before 1900 and 25 per cent have been built since 1945 as compared with 5 per cent in working class areas. In middle class areas as compared with working class areas more of the general practitioners had lists of less than 2,000 and fewer had lists with more than 2,500. Nearly twice as many of the general practitioners in the middle class areas had higher qualifications. More had access to contrast media X-rays. Nearly five times as many had access to physiotherapy. Twice as many held hospital appointments or had hospital beds into which they could admit their own patients.

Is There Anything We Can Do?

Of course there is much we can do. I have already discussed the redistribution of resources which is the major instrument which we must employ. If this is to be fully effective there are also questions of motivation and education within the service and its personnel. There is an increasing realization among health professionals of the kind of issues which I am discussing but there is need for further education. There is need of appropriate plans to deal with these circumstances and for dissemination of information and enthusiasm about the implementation of such plans. For example Baird in Aberdeen has demonstrated how the effectiveness of a carefully devised and vigorously executed programme in one area can be the stimulus to doing similar things elsewhere. Sometimes however a spread of improved practice even after demonstration may take considerable time. It has taken time to deploy the lessons from Baird's experience effectively in some parts of Scotland with the most adverse obstetric experience but this is now happening with beneficial results.

I have discussed the effect of fashion trends. There is no reason why we have to be passive in the face of this phenomenon. There are ways and means of accelerating the speed of movement of fashions down the social scale. This can be shown from differential experience with family planning. In communities where there has been a dynamic family planning programme the spread of family planning practices to lower social groups has been earlier and more rapid (Baird, 1975a).

There is need to recognize populations and individuals for whom normal National Health Service deployments are insufficient. The majority of those in greatest need are to be found concentrated in urban zones of general deprivation. Can we identify such zones and arrange that special provision is made for these zones with services appropriately provided and deployed to suit their circumstances? There will be need for study of appropriate indices on which to make such definitions, but we could already make rapid progress with existing information. We could for example draw upon the census study of areas of deprivation based on the Registrar General's enumeration districts (Department of the Environment, 1975). For a start the definition of enumeration districts within our towns in the 1 per cent or 5 per cent percentile of unemployment and overcrowding would give us in Scotland a valuable lead in defining zones for further examination. The definitions can be made more specific by addition of health service indicators. McIllwaine has demonstrated that mapping of wards in Glasgow in terms of such criteria as proportion of social class V and frequency of perinatal deaths sharply

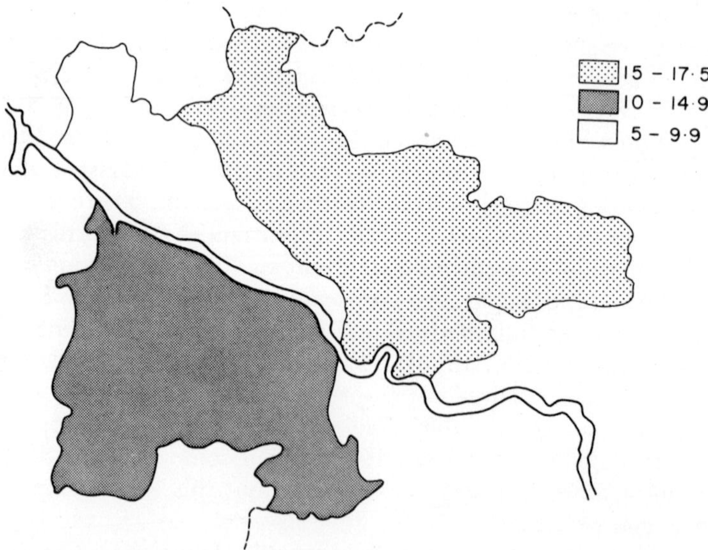

FIG. 13. Percentage resident male population (City of Glasgow) in social class V, by Ward, 1970. From McIllwaine (1974).

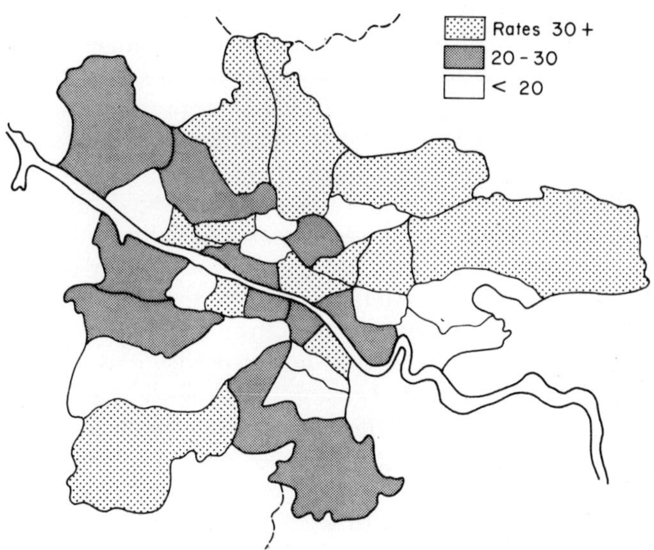

Fig. 14. City of Glasgow perinatal mortality rates by Ward, 1970. From McIlwaine (1974).

brings to notice those parts of the city in greatest need (McIllwaine, 1974). There is also an indication that these are often districts where service deployments are least effective.

The definition of target zones for specially devised efforts is probably the most effective way of meeting the needs of deprived families. But should we also attempt a definition and register of vulnerable families and individuals so that special efforts may be made on their behalf? If this is to be attempted it is necessary to be precise in our definition of families and individuals in need. This is much easier said than done. There is not only need to be specific but there is need to be restricted and restrained in the number of such families and individuals so defined. We are well aware of early experience with "at risk" registers for children where over-enthusiastic application of a variety of indices of risks led to definitions which embraced 50 per cent or more of the total child population. This kind of definition is self defeating. It is essential if we move into this specific targeting of families and individuals in need of help that we use definitions which produce limited and manageable numbers.

Douglas has recently suggested on the evidence of his studies that the single most identifying characteristic would be the time at which a mother presented for antenatal care (Douglas, 1971). A definition of the late-comers in his survey population identified a group with a high proportion of subsequent morbidities. For example those who came late for antenatal care made little use of child welfare and other services provided for them. This group included a large proportion of young mothers—and many who were rated by health visitors as giving unsatisfactory care to their infants. These mothers tended also to have closely placed births. They returned early to employment and their home conditions deteriorated in the succeeding year. Mortality of infants during the first four years of life was twice as high in this group of deficient users of antenatal services as in a matched group of those who had made good use of these services. Furthermore, 80 per cent of the deaths of children in such families occurred at home compared with only 10 per cent of the infant deaths in the matched groups. There were a number of other ways in which the children of the late attenders demonstrated greater serious morbidity.

There are other indices we could test out such as size of family, single parent families and families with a teenage mother especially where there had been pre-nuptial conception. With a combination of one or two indices of family demography and National Health Service behaviour it may be possible to identify a manageable population of high need clients.

Identification of families and individuals in this way is only the start of an essential but difficult process of turning round our methods of providing services for these people from "self-help" to "out-reach". There are many difficulties which must be overcome. There is the need to maintain information about the families some of whom will be urban nomads. There is the difficulty of establishing and maintaining contact in a practical and personal way with individuals who are suspicious of any kind of public service. There will be difficulty in recruiting workers with the capacity for stout-hearted as well as warm-hearted efforts in the face of rebuff and habits which run counter to the rules of well-regulated households. Any change of effort in this direction must be carried out in the full knowledge of difficulties. Radical change of deployments will require radical review of the consequences for methods of work. But already we have some evidence of what can be achieved by carrying services to even the most deprived families. This comes in part from the work of domiciliary family planning by Wilson and her colleagues in one of the most deprived parts of Glasgow. Not only has the birth rate there been halved, but new self-respect and health has been brought to mothers previously burdened with excessive child bearing (Wilson, 1971). We now have analogous although less dramatic evidence of the good effects from deploying a special health visiting effort for the children in a similar population; perhaps most encouraging of all is that the efforts are welcomed by the families involved.

In the broad area I have been discussing I am sure that everyone will agree there is great need for research. For example McKinlay draws our attention to the fact that whereas a considerable volume of study and investigation has demonstrated the association of greater mortality and morbidity and less efficient use of health services with certain social groups very little work has been done to study why there are these differences (McKinlay, 1969). We are indeed in great need of studies which can tell us more about the behaviour motivation and circumstances of vulnerable groups who are poor utilizers of service so that we can better understand how to redevise and redeploy our efforts. However, I think we must be careful that we do not use the cry for research as an alibi for present inactivity. There is much we can do with existing information—we should get ahead and do it. We should also encourage research to improve our later efforts.

References

Baird, D. (1969). An area maternity service. *Lancet*, **i**, 515–519.

Baird, D. (1973). Environmental factors in relation to obstetrics. In *Environmental Medicine*. Edited by G. M. Howe and J. A. Loraine. London: William Heinemann Medical Books.

Baird, D. (1974a). Epidemiology of congenital malformations of the central nervous system in (a) Aberdeen and (b) Scotland. *J. Biosoc. Sci.* **6**, 113–137.

Baird, D. (1974b). The epidemiology of low birth weight: changes in incidence in Aberdeen, 1948–72. *J. Biosoc. Sci.* **6**, 323–341.

Baird, D. (1975a). The changing pattern of human reproduction in Scotland, 1928–1972. *J. Biosoc. Sci.* **7**, 77–97.

Baird, D. (1975b). Interplay of changes in society, reproduction habits and obstetric practice in Scotland between 1922 and 1972. *Br. J. Prevent. Soc. Med.* **29**, 135.

Buchan, I. C. and Richardson, I. M. (1971). Time study of consultations in general practice. *Scottish Health Service Studies No.* **27**. Edinburgh: Scottish Home and Health Department.

Butler, N. R. and Bonham, D. G. (1963). *Perinatal Mortality*. Edinburgh and London: Livingstone.

Carstairs, V. and Patterson, P. E. (1966). Distribution of hospital patients by social class. *Hlth Bull.* **XXIV**, No. 3 (July).

Cartwright, A. (1964). *Human Relations and Hospital Care*. London: Routledge and Kegan Paul.

Cartwright, A. and Marshall, R. (1965). General practice in 1963. *Med. Care* **3**, 69.

Cartwright, A. and O'Brien, M. (1976). Social class variations in the nature of general practitioner consultations. In *Sociology of the NHS*. Edited by Margaret Stacey, Monograph No. 22. University of Keele, Staffs.

Central Statistical Office CSO(EBS) (10 July 1975). Editorial Board of "Social Trends", Social Commentary: Social Class.

Davie, R., Butler, V. and Goldstein, H. (1972). *From Birth to Seven.* London: Longman and The National Children's Bureau.

Department of the Environment (1975). *Census Indicators of Urban Deprivation.* Working Note 6, *Great Britain.* London: Department of the Environment.

Douglas, J. W. B. (1971). Personal communication. *Scottish Health Service Studies No.* **27.** Edinburgh: Scottish Home and Health Department.

Gordon, I. (1951). Social status and active prevention of disease. *Monthly Bull. Min. Hlth* **10**, 59–61.

Heasman, M. A. Problems of the National Health Service in Scotland today. (Unpublished paper.)

Illsley, R. (1955). Social class selection and class differences in relation to stillbirths and infant deaths. *Br. Med. J.* **ii**, 1520.

Illsley, R. (1967). The sociological study of reproduction and its outcome. In *Childbearing in its Social and Psychological Aspects.* Edited by S. A. Richardson and A. F. Guttmacher. New York: Williams and Wilkins.

Illsley, R. and Kincaid, J. C. (1963). Social correlations of perinatal mortality. In *Perinatal Mortality.* Edited by N. R. Butler and D. G. Bonham. Edinburgh and London: Livingstone.

Logan, W. P. D. (1960). *Morbidity Statistics from General Practice* Vol. 2. *Occupations.* General Register Office: Studies on Medical and Population Subjects, No. 14. London: Her Majesty's Stationery Office.

MacGregor, J. E. and Baird, D. (1963). Detection of cervical carcinoma in the general population. *Br. Med. J.* **i**, 1631.

McIllwaine, G. M. (1974). *Social and Obstetric Factors in Relation to Perinatal Mortality in Glasgow.* PhD Thesis, University of Glasgow.

McKinlay, J. B. (1969). Comment on class attitudes to dental treatment. *Br. J. Sociol.* **20**, 85–87.

McKinlay, J. B. (1970). Research report. A brief description of a study on the utilisation of maternity and child welfare services by a lower working class subculture. *Social Sci. Med.* **4**, 551–556.

McKinlay, J. B. and McKinlay, S. (1972). Some social characteristics of lower working class utilizers and underutilizers of maternity care services. *J. Hlth Soc. Behav.* **13**, 369–382.

Nelignan, G., Prudham, D. and Steiner, H. (1974). *The Formative Years.* London: Oxford University Press and The Nuffield Trust.

Office of Population Censuses and Surveys (1975). *General Household Survey*, 1972. London: Her Majesty's Stationery Office.

Rein, M. (1969). Social class and the utilization of medical care services, Hospitals. *J. Am. Hlth Assoc.* **43** (July).

Richards, I. D. G. (1971). *Infant Mortality in Scotland.* Scottish Health Service Studies No. 27. Edinburgh: Scottish Home and Health Department.

Titmuss, R. M. (1969). *Commitment to Welfare.* London: George Allen and Unwin.

Which (1975). The National Health Service: How well does it work? August.

Wilson, E. (1971). Domiciliary family planning service in Glasgow. *Br. Med. J.* **iv**, 731–733.

How Doctors Generate Disease

DONALD GOULD

The New Statesman, London, England

Doctors are generally held in awe and respect by a majority of their fellow citizens because of wishful thinking. People desperately want to believe that there is a remedy for every human ill, and even a way of cheating death. Doctors are the agents through whom these hopes just might be fulfilled, and they are therefore invested, in the imagination of the populace, with supernormal wisdom and powers, just as the priest is so regarded by those hoping for the favour of God and a ticket of admission to Eternal Life.

It is, of course, true that doctors can now relieve a great deal of physical suffering, and can often postpone death. But the gratitude and wonderment which these abilities generate among their customers tend to prevent a recognition of the fact that the medical profession may be as potent a cause for evil as for good. People just do not want to know about the grimy side of the coin.

The true importance of the medical profession to the health of nations may be crudely judged by two examples. For over a quarter of a century Britain's National Health Service has made expert medical care available to all at the time of need without charge, and yet over the past 20 years the time lost from work due to sickness has increased nationwide by a prodigious 24 per cent. During a doctors' strike in the Canadian province of Saskatchewan some 13 years ago when treatment was only available for the desperately ill in two or three hospitals specially staffed by the warring doctors for the purpose, no single death occurred which was attributable to the unavailability of instant medical care. Indeed, the province's mortality figures actually fell below the average for the time of year.

The greatest damage doctors do to their patients involves the misuse of drugs. Excessive and over-enthusiastic treatment is by no means a new phenomenon. Louis XIII is said to have suffered 212 enemas, 215 purgations and 47 bleedings within the course of a single year, and a canon of Troyes was once sued for the cost of 2,190 enemas administered to him over a period of two years. However, the major virtue of the therapies of the past is that if few did those subjected to them any good, most of them did not do all that much damage either.

Modern drugs have created an entirely different situation. Their very value depends upon the fact that they are capable of altering the biochemistry of cells and organs. It therefore follows that no effective drug can be innocuous. If it can alter the body chemistry in some desired fashion it must also, either incidentally or because of misuse, be capable of producing undesirable, or dangerous, or fatal effects.

In view of the fact that the great majority of human ills are now treated (at least by the practitioners of orthodox Western medicine) with the powerful synthetic chemicals produced by the pharmaceutical industry, it is astounding, as well as dangerous and deplorable, that the training of a doctor includes virtually no instruction in the manner in which modern remedies should be handled, or what a drug may be expected to accomplish, or how to assess whether that expectation is fulfilled.

Doctors belong to a most conservative profession within which attitudes change at a painfully slow pace, and senior physicians, still in active practice, were trained at a time when no more than a handful of effective remedies existed (drugs like quinine, digitalis, insulin and morphine). Therefore the emphasis in clinical teaching and, indeed, the chief interest of the practicing doctor lay in the business of diagnosis and prognosis. Treatment was almost an afterthought, and the sections on treatment in the medical textbooks were commonly both brief and filled with vague platitudes such as "Attention should be pakd to the bowels," or "Adequate rest should be ensured by the administration of sedatives as required". Despite the major change brought about by the therapeutic revolution, pride of place is still given to diagnostic skills and techniques. The therapeutic tools which modern doctors use have been almost entirely the product of research undertaken by the pharmaceutical industry. They have not been evolved by the doctors who use them. A majority of general practitioners and, probably, a good many hospital doctors, rely for their knowledge of drug therapy on the literature supplied by the manufacturers.

The result of all this is that Sir Ronald Bodley Scott, the chairman of the Medicines Commission, can say

> Doctors of my generation, particularly those in general practice (because hospital doctors do not pick up a certain amount of information) have no idea how to use, I suppose, 90 per cent of modern drugs.

And a High Street dispensing chemist—a past president of the Pharmaceutical Society has recently described the prescribing habits of family doctors as "diabolical". He tells the story of an elderly man who came to him with a prescription for digoxin. The man had been on the drug for three years and had obtained supplies from other chemists on repeat prescriptions. But this time the pharmacist noticed that the old chap had been prescribed three times the usual dose. Digoxin, which affects the activity of the heart muscle, is a dangerous poison at too high a dose, and the margin between an effective and a dangerous dose is small. The chemist therefore rang up the doctor concerned, and queried the prescription. The doctor said "Oh, God! I remember him. He was only supposed to be on three tablets a day for the first week. Change it to one a day, will you?"

Professor James Crooks of the Department of Pharmacology and Therapeutics at Dundee, one of the very few medical scientists in the country specializing in the study of drug use and misuse, holds that even heart specialists often use digoxin improperly. They think they know what they are doing, he says, but since they qualified a great deal of laboratory work on the action of digoxin has taken place which they are unaware. They see their patients, and commit them to a long-term course of digoxin therapy, and often these patients develop symptoms of poisoning. But then they come under the care of a geriatrician, and the clever heart specialist never sees the results of his inept therapy.

Professor Crooks says that in his part of the world 30 per cent of hospital patients suffer some kind of unwanted effect from the drugs they are given, and in 5 per cent of patients entering hospital a drug has contributed to the illness necessitating the admission.

He is particularly concerned at the manner in which old people are often prescribed a whole range of powerful medicines for the various failings of the flesh common to old age. He tells the story of one old lady who recently came under his care. At various times she had been put on continuing doses of thyroxine, digoxin, a diuretic, potassium tablets and a hypnotic. She could not possibly sort all this out. She simply knew that she had to take five tablets at a go. She put all her various pills in one container and shook out the appropriate number whenever medicine time came round. One day she happened to shake out five digoxin tablets, and was soon after admitted to hospital with acute digoxin poisoning. Professor Crooks calls this game, which is very commonly played by old people, pharmacological Russian roulette.

A bright and critically minded young doctor working in a London teaching hospital describes his discomfort at a tendency displayed by some of the keen and "scientifically minded" super-specialists with whom he comes in contact. They give dangerous drugs to correct some esoteric aberration in body chemistry discovered during the course of intensive and blanket laboratory investigations. The "fault" may not have been causing the patient the smallest distress. This same young doctor describes a routine practised in his own unit. "When a patient is looking really ill and we're not quite sure what to do we sometimes withdraw *all* medication for 24 hours and see what happens. Sometimes patients who've been dull and drowsy and apparently on the way to death do come round. Then you realize the horrific fact that you've been poisoning them."

Chronic and acute poisoning from drugs prescribed for the relief of physical or mental distress is probably far commoner than most of us realize. A UK study in 1969 suggested that over half of all British adults and almost a third of British children take some kind of medication every day, and 75 per cent of the medicines swallowed are obtained on repeat prescriptions, a high proportion of which will probably have been issued without the doctor concerned having re-examined or even spoken to the patient. Under these circumstances it would be reasonable to suppose that at any one time some millions of UK citizens are suffering from some degree of adverse drug reaction.

The ignorant and irresponsible use of modern drugs is the most obvious but by no means the only way in which doctors generate disease. They sometimes make unimportant or even entirely imaginary ailments matters for fashionable concern. The celebrated British surgeon, Sir Arbuthnot Lane, who died as recently as 1943 put forward the proposition, entirely without supporting evidence, that many of the ills of the flesh arise from poisons absorbed into the blood stream from the faecal contents of the large intestine. Employing a kind of mad logic he cut out the colons of over a thousand trusting customers in an attempt to relieve them of the probably imagined symptoms produced by the certainly imaginary toxins they were supposed to be absorbing.

More recently other surgical exercises of dubious value have been in vogue. In the 1930s between a half and three quarters of all British children had their tonsils ripped out, often in bloody and painful "production-line" sessions. Apart from the totally unnecessary pain and suffering caused to the unfortunate victims of this surgical ritual, and the not infrequent tragic death from uncontrollable bleeding, an American study (in the days before mass polio immunization) revealed that after tonsillectomy children ran a fourfold increased risk of developing bulbar poliomyelitis. And much more recently (in 1971) another study has shown that people without their tonsils are three times more likely to develop Hodgkin's disease.

Psychosurgery has come in for increasing criticism by people who regard this particular effort at relieving the symptoms of mental disease as an unjustifiable assault on the personality and even the soul of the patient concerned. Perhaps psychosurgery has made a previously intolerable situation bearable for some, but there is also little doubt that profligate and irresponsible use of this technique has caused damaging personality changes in many patients without any compensating improvement in their original intellectual defect. Then there are the strangely called "heroic" surgeons who undertake the most drastic feats of biological engineering, such as heart and liver transplants, more, it sometimes seems, for the glory of achieving a technical triumph than because their efforts offer any great prospect of reducing the sum of human suffering. Despite a few "successes" the heart transplant enthusiasts have clearly caused a great deal more pain, discomfort and distress than they have been able to relieve.

Apart from damage to individual patients, doctors have also been responsible for some dangerous tampering with nature of a kind which may prove disastrous to society as a whole. Take only two examples. A massive reduction of deaths from infections such as malaria, in the absence of any policy for adequately feeding and housing and employing the many millions whose lives have been saved, has contributed significantly to the population explosion, and the increasingly bitter competition for a share of the world's strictly finite natural resources, and this situation is the one which might lead, within decades, to a true and final Armageddon. But supposing that, as a result of a series of so-far unforeseeable political and technological miracles, the species is spared for a few more centuries, then (some entirely sober-minded scientists argue) medicine's increasing capacity to keep alive the mentally and physically unfit will so interfere with the process of natural selection, and will so corrupt the genetic pool, that the species *Homo sapiens* will degenerate, and be beaten in the struggle for survival.

Many would mock at these last two predictions of disaster, regarding them as the vapourings of a doomwatcher's fevered imagination. Be that as it may, none can deny the modern doctor's increasing powers for doing great harm as well as immense good. It is perhaps time to divert some of the energy and high intelligence and expertise at present aimed at advancing medical science and technology to the equally
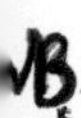
important and urgent task of deciding how best the skills we already possess can be used to improve, and not to damage, Man's estate.

Social Class and Health Inequalities

M. BLAXTER

Institute of Medical Sociology, Aberdeen, Scotland

A sociologist faced with the task of discussing social class and health inequalities is placed in a dilemma. If inequalities are to be demonstrated in an unequivocal way, it is necessary to talk in terms of a very simple class structure. The dividing-up and labelling of the various strata of society has been a popular pursuit ever since the days when Charles Booth devised an eight-fold division of the population of London, ranging from the 18 per cent of "middle-class" at the top to the 1 per cent of "loafers, drunkards and semi-criminals" at the bottom. Our current system, based on occupational status, rejects these moral overtones but still raises many problems and contains many anomalies. This is inevitable, for the attempt to divide a changing society into a handful of more or less self-contained strata that form an hierarchical order manifestly does violence to the infinite complexity of human relationships. In particular, it has to be asked what relevance it has to the experiences of the individuals so pigeon-holed. Increasingly, research appears to show that awareness of inequality is complex, perception of deprivation is relative, and what appears from the outside to be homogenous is, when viewed from the inside, highly differentiated.

Thus, a sociologist is reluctant to use any simple social classification. And yet, having said all this, one is faced with the straightforward facts that Sir John Brotherston has reviewed in the Galton Lecture: the fact that there are seemingly intractible class differentials in perinatal mortality, the fact that physical inequalities at birth still widen between classes as the babies become children (Miller *et al.*, 1974), the fact that, although every cause of death has its own pattern, overall mortality rates still rise regularly from social class I to social class V.

Social class, therefore, does mean something. To examine these persistent differentials more closely, discussion will first be centred on mortality figures. An attempt will then be made to link these to what is known about morbidity, and lastly morbidity will be related to the use of health services, seeking clues at each stage which may hint at explanations for the stage before.

For these purposes it is necessary to talk in broad statistical terms. I should hope, eventually, to return to a consideration of what social class really means, but to begin with the evidence must be offered in simple terms of the Registrar General's social classes.

The Evidence about Mortality

So, turning first to statistics of mortality, the standard and optimistic story of social class differentials goes something like this. In the bad old days when access to medical care was unequal, and environmental causes of ill-health were very prominent, social class differentials could not but be expected to be great. Now that medical science and social conscience have both advanced, and some of these environmental causes have been tackled, death rates from many diseases—the "old" diseases of poverty—have tumbled. Mortality from tuberculosis is less than a quarter of what it was 30 years ago; deaths of middle-age men from pneumonia have more than halved since sulphonamides. Cities are still unhealthy, but not longer quite as unhealthy as they were in 1854 when Snow looked into the Southwark and Vauxhall Company's water supply and condemned the Broad Street pump.

Inasmuch as inborn and environmental inequalities remain, social class differences in these "old" diseases very directly influenced by infection and poor environment, may be expected to persist, but they are lessening as society becomes more equal and the benefits of modern public health and scientific medicine become, in Britain, free to all. On the other hand, there are the "new" diseases, the diseases of affluence, which used to have a negative social class gradient—the diseases associated with obesity, the business executive's coronary. We may expect this gradient to slacken, as the "benefits" of affluence spread through the population.

What, in fact, is happening?

Figure 1 gives, as a starting-point, a simple representation of the way in which mortality rates of men varied by social class for the latest period for which such an analysis is available, 1959–63. It is perhaps illuminating to consider different age-groups: three examples are shown, in all of which the deaths might be termed unnecessary deaths, deaths before old age. A slackening of the social class gradient as men get older is of course to be expected, since those men who survive are by definition healthier, although there is also a process which might be

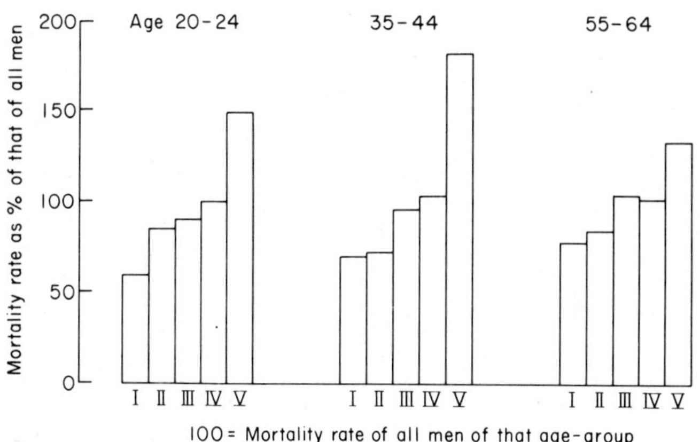

FIG. 1. Mortality rates by social class. Men, 1959–63, three age-groups, England and Wales (*Registrar General*, 1971).

expected to counteract this: the occupational mobility upwards and downwards during their lifetimes of the more and less healthy.

As Brotherston has pointed out, it is difficult to find evidence that these social class differences in mortality are at present lessening. Indeed, the Registrar General's report of 1971 on occupational mortality commented that one of the most disturbing features was that, even when adjustments had been made for changes in the classification system and changes in the relative sizes of classes, there was a social class V group whose position had apparently deteriorated and who "did not benefit from the considerable benefits of the decade as did the majority of their compatriots". In order to examine this apparent widening of class differentials more closely, different groups of diseases may be examined.

Figure 2 shows the contribution made by some of the "old" diseases, the diseases of poverty, to these apparent overall trends. While rates of mortality from these diseases have fallen steeply, the difference between classes appears to have widened. Widening differentials can be explained, in an increasingly mobile society, by the operation of a more efficient selection process, though it is easier to accept this as the whole explanation at the bottom of the class scale than it is at the top.

What of "diseases of affluence"? It was expected that, as affluence spread, so should these diseases—but Fig. 3 shows examples of gradients which have in fact completely reversed. There are now very few diseases indeed where the rates in social classes I and II are higher than those in classes IV and V.

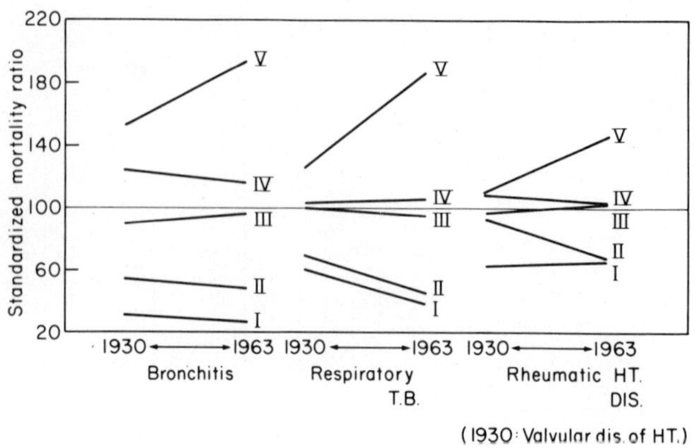

Fig. 2. Some "old" diseases: trends of mortality ratios. Men, 1930–63, ages 15–64, England and Wales (*Registrar General*, 1971).

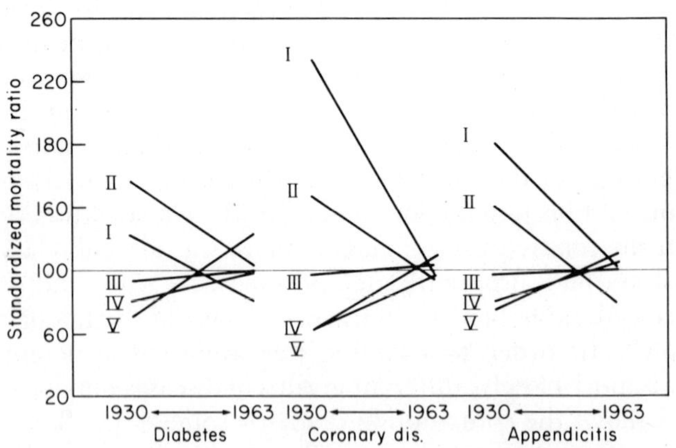

Fig. 3. Some "new" diseases: trends of mortality ratios. Men, 1930–63, ages 15–64, England and Wales (*Registrar General*, 1971).

Mortality is not, of course, the same as morbidity: death rates do not necessarily tell us everything about health. Before leaving mortality statistics, however, there is one more example which not only underlines the point already made but serves as a link between mortality, morbidity and service use. Figure 4 shows the trends of mortality over 30 years for some of the cancers: breast and cervical cancer in married women, and cancer of the stomach and prostate in men. Remembering

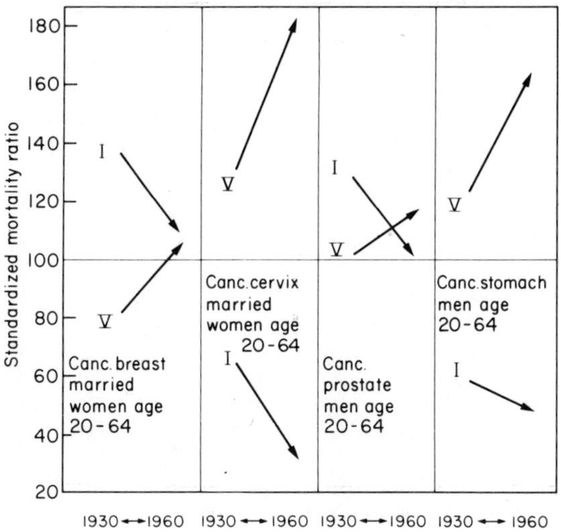

FIG. 4. Certain cancers: trends of mortality ratios, 1930–60, England and Wales, social classes I and V (*Registrar General*, (1971).

that we are talking about deaths before old age, these are diseases where early identification and treatment are important. For simplicity, only classes I and V are compared. In those cancers which have always been commonest in the lower classes, the differential has increased, and for those which used to have a negative social class gradient, the differential has tended towards reversal. Mortality rates were of course falling during this period for cervical and stomach cancer, as they were for the "diseases of poverty", and rising for cancer of the breast and (to a lesser extent) prostate. It appears to be the rule, to which there are very few exceptions, that where rates are falling class differentials are widening, and where they are rising, differentials reverse. It is hard to escape the conclusion that in conditions where medical science is making great strides, there is a cultural lag in the diffusion of these advances throughout the social classes.

The Evidence about Morbidity

It must be repeated that it is theoretically possible for death-rates to tell us little about the distribution of ill-health, for it may be that there are concealed differences between groups in the seriousness of the disease or the success of its treatment. Of course, we simply do not know how much ill-health exists. We have statistics for hospitals, and for a

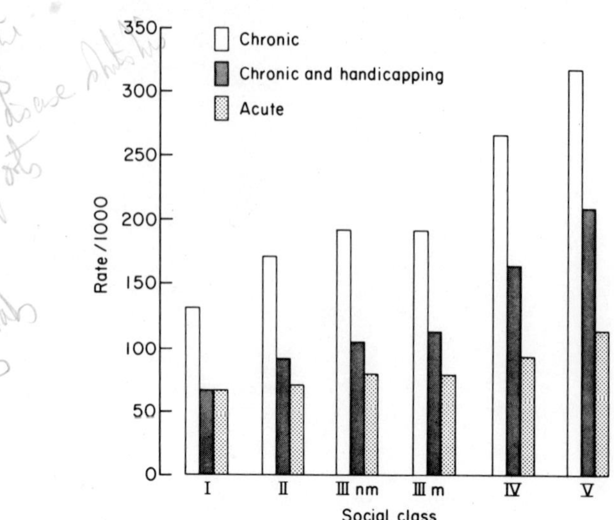

FIG. 5. Rates of self-reported illness by social class, per 1,000 people, men and women, all ages, Great Britain (*General Household Survey*, 1972).

small number of individual diseases, but for the general run of illness treated in the community—or, of course, not treated at all—there is only the evidence of surveys in which the extent of illness declared is self-reported, and open to question as a precise measure. Aware as we all are of our own hypochondria, it is natural that a first reaction is to assume that perhaps people exaggerate. The relationship of self-reported health status to clinically-defined disease is a complex area of study, but the many studies that have compared self-reported illness with clinical examination have found without exception that disease is under-reported, usually greatly (Pearse and Crocker, 1954; Krueger, 1957; Cartwright, 1959; Kosa *et al.*, 1967. See also Mechanic and Newton, 1965; Haberman, 1969). It would, of course, be relevant if there were a consistent social class variation in the self-reporting of illness. The major evidence comes from the United States (Breslow, 1957; Commission on Chronic Illness, 1959; US National Center for Health Statistics, 1965), and there are of course problems about extrapolating from another country which uses different social classifications and has a different structure of medical care. However, these studies confirm more limited ones in this country to show less reporting of clinically-found illness in lower social classes, which would indicate that the trends shown in Fig. 5 are likely, if anything, to be an understatement.

Figure 5 shows the amounts of illness reported in the General Household Survey, according to social classes. These rates are for all ages, and both sexes, and may conceal differences between men and women which will be considered later. Three types of illness are considered: acute, chronic, and handicapping, which asks of those with chronic illnesses "Does it limit your activities compared with most people of your own age?" and acute, which is the answer to the question whether there was any illness or injury which restricted normal activity during a two-week reference period. Dividing reported illness in this way at least gives some indication of what we are choosing that the word should mean.

It can be seen that differences in mortality are at least paralleled by differences in morbidity, and the difference occurs in chronic rather than acute illness. Even if examination is confined to the more stringent and objective condition of handicapping chronic illness, prevalence rates in social class V, at over 200 per 1,000 people, are well over twice the rate of 75 reported in class I.

The next step is to place this experience of morbidity against mortality. Figure 6 shows rates of handicapping chronic illness and acute illness expressed as percentage deviations from the average experience of all people in a particular sex/age group, set besides mortality expressed in the same way. Here two age groups are distinguished and the sexes separated, and for simplicity only social classes and I are V compared.

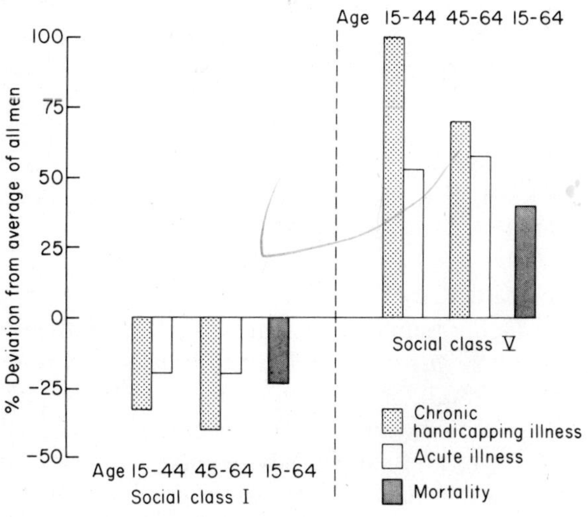

Fig. 6. Rates of illness compared with mortality—men: special classes I and V.

The argument has been put forward, principally by Professor Martin Rein (1969), that class mortality is not an index of class morbidity. This evidence suggests that, on the contrary, the difference in morbidity is greater than mortality figures would suggest. A second point which this comparison shows is that the excess morbidity in social class V occurs at younger ages rather than in late middle age.

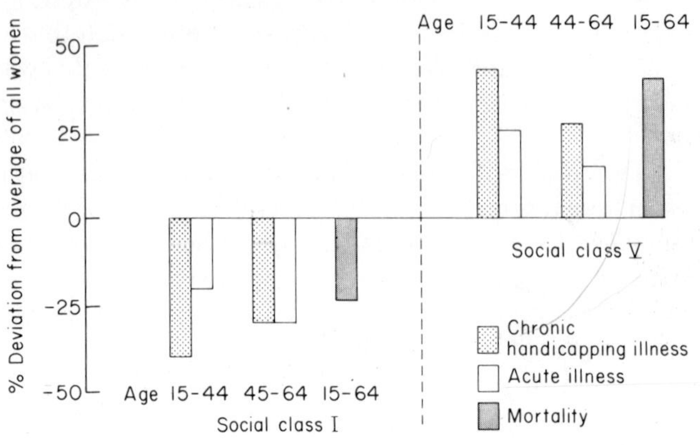

FIG. 7. Rates of illness compared with mortality—women: social classes I and V.

In Figure 7 the comparisons between morbidity and mortality are repeated for women, and it is evident that social class differences, though still real, are much less extreme for women. The reasons for this are a matter for speculation, though it must be noted that the definitions of illness being used involve some idea of handicap or restricted activity, and it may be that there is less social class difference among women in the way that they define what "normal" activity is. It is also true that the fact of assortive mating, combined with the fact that married women are categorized by their husband's occupational class, would lead one to expect less social class variation among women.

The Evidence of Health-Care Statistics

The intervening factor between mortality and morbidity is of course medical care: one may suffer many illnesses but receive good treatment and recover from them all, or one may suffer few illnesses but nevertheless be more likely to die because of poorer care. Leaving aside a privileged few, too few to matter statistically, we like to think that the availability of medical care in this country is irrespective of social class. The ways in which this can be measured are limited. Questions can, however, be asked about the use made of medical services.

Figure 8 shows, for instance, the average number of reported consultations per person/per year with a general practitioner, for different social classes, for men and for women, and for three different age groups. These figures are again from the General Household Survey, and on the whole they are in agreement with other sources of consultation statistics (e.g. Cartwright, 1967; Royal College of General Practitioners, 1973; Logan and Cushion, 1974).

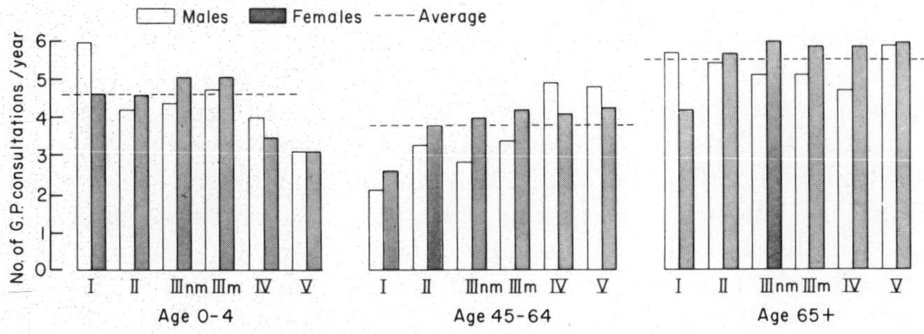

FIG. 8. Number of general practitioner consultations (N.H.S.) by social class, per person per year, three age groups, Great Britain (General Household Survey, 1972).

Three groups are shown to illustrate how interestingly patterns vary at different ages. Over 65, it would appear that social class differences in the use of primary medical care largely disappear. For infants, there is a conspicuous falling-off in general practitioner consultations in the semi- and unskilled groups. (Incidentally, the remarkable difference between male and female infants in social class I is supported by other evidence as being a real one. Male infants are, of course, slightly less healthy, statistically speaking, than female: nevertheless for the majority of the population, classes II and III, more use is made of primary care for female infants.) Clinics are, of course, an alternative source of primary care for infants. Unfortunately, there is much evidence to show that they too are under-used, proportionately, by the lowest social classes (McKinlay, 1972).

The patterns at ages 45–64 (and this group is chosen so that women's childbearing years do not complicate the picture) show a fairly regular rise as social class declines: whereas males in social classes I and II consult general practitioners on average two or three times a year, in social class IV and V it is four or five times. These differences may seem small, but if a difference of nearly 100 per cent is translated into number of general practitioners required, they fall into perspective. One other point worthy of note is the sex difference: whereas in classes I to III manual, the classes in which poverty is not widespread, women use their general practitioners more than men, the reverse is true of the wives of semi- and unskilled men.

We have already seen, however, that the lower social classes *need* more medical help than the higher: the evidence from both mortality and morbidity is that they suffer more illnesses. The next obvious question is how these match, proportionately. Do lower social classes use medical services, and in particular general practitioners, to an extent greater than their greater ill-health would warrant? It is not unknown for some general practitioners to make this suggestion.

As a test of this, a "consultation index" has been calculated. For each group, this is obtained by dividing the consultation rate/1,000 people (in a two-week period) by the amount of illness they reported. Which of the available definitions of illness is used is a matter of choice. One might use reported acute illness, which varies least between classes, or chronic illness, which varies most. I have chosen to use the middle measure, the reported prevalence of chronic illness which the patient claims actually restricts him in the activities of daily life. This is the more interesting measure, since it involves a greater element of choice about consulting a doctor than an acute illness, and it is also less influenced by any tendency to define restricted activity by whether or not one required a certificate of incapacity for work, which will obviously have a social class component.

TABLE I

Consultation Indices

Comparing the prevalence of chronic handicapping illness with general practitioner and hospital outpatient consultation rates

Social class	General practitioner index[a]		Hospital outpatient index[b]	
	M	F	M	F
I	1·20	2·03	1·29	1·56
II	1·04	1·34	0·99	1·08
IIInm	0·91	1·29	1·02	1·05
IIIm	0·84	1·20	0·93	0·84
IV	0·75	0·76	0·66	0·58
V	0·59	0·69	0·63	0·49

Data from General Household Survey, 1972.

[a] Rate per 1,000 people of general practitioner consultations in a two-week period /prevalence rate per 1,000 people of chronic handicapping illness.

[b] Rate per 1,000 people of hospital outpatient consultation in a three-month period/prevalence rate per 1,000 people of chronic handicapping illness.

Table I shows without doubt that although the lower social classes may use their general practitioners more in terms of simple number, the higher social classes use them more in relation to the amount of illness they perceive themselves as suffering. For every visit that a man in social class V who has a chronic illness pays to his doctor, a man in social class I pays two, and for women the difference is even more marked. These indices are for all ages, and may conceal differences between age-groups. If all the figures for different age-groups are calculated, patterns emerge which I can only summarize: for men, the apparent under-use is particularly marked in the children of the manual classes, and in younger adults in social class V. For women, relative under-use is prominent in the three manual classes at all adult ages before 64, but less marked in children and the elderly.

Simple numbers of consultations are not, of course, the whole story: it is necessary to consider their content as well as their quantity. This is not a question very amenable to statistical investigation, but there is persuasive evidence that, as Titmuss claimed in 1968, "the higher income groups know how to make better use of the Health Service". There is evidence, for instance, that middle class consultations have a higher clinical content, and working-class a higher administrative one; working-class people tend to have doctors with larger lists than middle-class patients, and professional people are likely to have doctors with what are assumed to be advantageous characteristics—those who hold hospital appointments, for instance, or who are more recently qualified (Cartwright, 1967). A recent study (Marsh and McNay, 1974) investigating the use of all the members of the medical team in a large general practice found that the resources of the team as a whole, including for instance the services of the Health Visitor, were used most by social classes I and II.

This is primary medical care: what of specialist care? A similar index can be calculated for hospital outpatient consultations, and in the slide it is compared with the general practitioner index. It is perhaps a little disturbing to find—since here we are approaching doctor-defined illness rather than self-defined; no-one obtains an outpatient consultation unless a doctor has considered it necessary—that virtually the same gradient appears. For every one consultation in social class V, there are 2 for men and 3 for women in social class I. The sharp drop between the skilled on the one hand, and the semi- and unskilled workers on the other, is again prominent: it seems uncontrovertible that women, particularly, in the lowest social classes are receiving less than their share of medical care.

Other evidence about the use of services may be noted briefly. It is well known, for instance, that there is a social class gradient in preventive medicine (Weeks, 1958; Rosenstock, 1969; Suchman, 1965). Some of the clearest evidence comes from the National Child Development Survey (Davie, 1972) from which some very sad statistics can be extracted which connect medical need and use of services in a particularly direct way. At seven years old, it seems from Table II that the relationship between clinically-defined need for specialist services (a need with profound consequences for the children's future) and the use of these services, was clear—and, for the most part, inverse.

TABLE II
Need and service utilization
Percentage of seven-year-old children who:

	Social class					
	I	II	IIInm	IIIm	IV	V
Had poor dental health (10 or more DMF teeth)	6·5	8·8	10·0	9·7	11·4	9·6
Had ever attended dental clinic, dentist or orthodontist	83·3	79·9	80·9	76·2	72·5	67·6
Had not fully intelligible speech	5·5	8·4	9·5	14·9	18·3	22·1
Had ever attended for speech therapy	2·8	2·0	2·1	2·4	2·8	3·0
Had signs of past or present otitis media	6·8	5·8	7·7	7·4	6·8	9·6
Had ever attended a hearing or audiology clinic	8·6	7·0	7·9	7·7	7·6	7·1

National Child Development Survey, 1965.

Conclusions

If, as I hope I have shown, social class inequalities persist not only in health but also in health care, what remedies can be suggested? It can be argued that inequality is inevitable. Inasmuch as people are being categorized into social classes on a scale involving, in a complex way, such factors as occupational risks, education, income, living environment, we are in a sense creating inequalities in health: we cannot pretend to be surprised if the top and the bottom of the scale differ. The amount of difference depends on the economic and political structure of a given society.

The point to which I have been moving, however, is this: we have a very complex and expensive structure in our society which has the function of correcting the variation as far as possible. It is not suggested that in an advanced society medical services are the main determinant of mortality and morbidity: obviously the causes of inequality lie primarily elsewhere. In an ideal society, however, the greatest need would be matched by the highest standard of service, so that these inequalities might be compensated for as far as possible.

There is perhaps a widening gap between modern medicine, committed to a highly scientific approach, and large sections of the lay public. Attempts to close the gap with new forms of service or with "health education" must be conceived in terms which are meaningful to the patients, for whom the problems of everyday living may be much more real than the postponed rewards of preventive medicine. There are many groups of the population whose position in the social structure makes it difficult for them to subscribe to that belief in the rational mastery of the world which typifies the professional approach: for them, the focus has to be on adjustment rather than control. A phrase from a survey of my own lingers in my mind: it was spoken by a middle-aged woman of social class V, a neglected and rapidly-deteriorating diabetic. She summed up her life by saying—"Oh, well, it can't be helped, it's a lucky person who has good health." This seemed to me to epitomize the attitude of resignation that was the fruit of a lifetime's inequalities.

But in this age, and in this society, it ought not to be just a matter of "luck". To change these attitudes, it may be that we ought to reconsider the structure of medical care. Perhaps our medicine is too scientific, too professional. Other countries have found it practicable to have a tier of more accessible, less highly-qualified, medical workers able to deal perfectly efficiently with much routine illness. Might it be that we ought to *welcome* dilution in medical education? Or that we need more *women* doctors? Or perhaps that we need not more doctors but more health visitors, district nurses, medical and psychiatric social workers, and with more responsibility. Almost certainly, we need to resist the temptation to strive after marginal and exciting improvements at ever-increasing cost, at the expense of consolidation at a more mundane level. Particularly at a time when financial stringency is in the air, we need clear thinking and wide-ranging public discussion about priorities. This need arises, however, not only from escalating costs but also, as Sir George Godber (1970) has pointed out, from the greater effectiveness of modern medicine, which provides an ever-widening range of real choices.

It is generally agreed that our distribution of medical resources matches ill with the social and geographical distribution of mortality and morbidity: this has been summed up by Hart (1975) with but slight exaggeration as the inverse care law: "the availability of good medical care tends to vary inversely with the need of the population served". If, however, we are really serious about reducing social class inequalities in health, then I suggest that we must, on the contrary, provide positive discrimination in favour of the greatest need.

References

Breslow, L. (1957). Uses and limitations of the California Health Survey studying the epidemiology of chronic disease. *Amer. J. Publ. Hlth* **47**, 168.

Cartwright, A. (1959). Problems in the collection and analysis of morbidity data. *Milbank Mem. Fund Quart.* **37**, 33.

Cartwright, A. (1967). *Patients and Their Doctors.* London: Routledge and Kegan Paul.

Commission on Chronic Illness (1959). *Chronic Illness in a Large City.* Cambridge, Mass.: Harvard University Press.

Davie, R. (1972). *From Birth to Seven: The Second Report of the National Child Development Survey* (**1958** *Cohort*). London: Longman and the National Children's Bureau.

Godber, Sir George (1970). *J. Roy. Coll. Gen. Practit.* **20**, 313.

Haberman, P. W. (1969). The reliability and validity of the data. In *Poverty and Health*, p. 343. Edited by J. Kosa, A. Antonovsky and I. Zola. Cambridge, Mass.: Harvard University Press.

Hart, J. T. (1975). The inverse care law. In *A Sociology of Medical Practice.* Edited by C. Cox and A. Mead. London: Collier-Macmillan.

Kosa, J., Alpert, J. J. and Haggerty, R. J. (1967). On the reliability of family health information. *Soc. Sci. Med.* **1**, 165.

Krueger, D. E. (1957). Measurement of prevalence of chronic disease by household interviews and clinical evaluations. *Amer. J. Publ. Hlth*, **47**, 953.

Logan, W. P. D. and Cushion, A. A. (1974). *Morbidity Statistics from General Practice, Second National Study* **1970–71**. Studies on Medical and Population Subjects No. 26, O.P.C.S. London: Her Majesty's Stationery Office.

McKinlay, J. B. (1972). Utilisers and underutilisers of maternity care systems. *J. Hlth Soc. Behav.* **13**, 4.

Marsh, G. N. and McNay, R. M. (1974). Team work load in an English general practice. *Br. Med. J.* **i**, 5903, 315.

Mechanic, D. and Newton, Margaret (1965). Some problems in the analysis of morbidity data. *J. Chron. Dis.* **18**, 569.

Miller, F. J. W., Court, S. D. M., Knox, E. G. and Brandon, S. (1974). *The School Years in Newcastle upon Tyne* **1952–62**. London: Oxford University Press.

Office of Population Censuses and Surveys (1975). *General Household Survey*, **1972**. London: Her Majesty's Stationery Office.

Pearse, I. H. and Crocker, L. H. (1954). *The Peckham Experiment.* London: George Allen and Unwin.

Registrar General (1971). *Decennial Supplement, England and Wales*, **1961**, *Occupational Mortality Tables.* London: Her Majesty's Stationery Office.

Rein, M. (1969). *J. Amer. Hosp. Assoc.* **43**; and *New Society*, 20 Nov., 807.

Rosenstock, I. M. (1969). Prevention of illness and maintenance of health. In *Poverty and Health*, p. 168. Edited by J. Kosa, A. Antonovsky and I. Zola. Cambridge, Mass.: Harvard University Press.

Royal College of General Practitioners (1973). *Present State and Future Needs of General Practice.* Reports from *General Practice*, No. 16. London.

Suchman, E. A. (1965). Social factors in medical deprivation. *Am. J. Publ. Hlth*, **55**, 1725.

Titmuss, R. M. (1968). *Commitment to Welfare*. London: George Allen and Unwin.

US National Center for Health Statistics (1965). *Health Interview Responses Compared with Medical Records*. Public Health Service Publication 1000, Series 2, No. 7.

Weeks, H. A. (1958). Apathy of families toward medical care. In *Patients, Physicians and Illness*. Edited by J. E. Gartly. New York: Free Press of Glencoe.

Urban and Suburban Differentials

R. J. DONALDSON

Centre for Extension Training in Community Medicine, London, England

Introduction

A number of contributions to this volume have dealt with the geographical distribution of disease and health inequalities on the macro scale. This paper deals with health inequalities on the micro scale.

The study was carried out in the County Borough of Teesside where I was Medical Officer of Health from its formation in 1968 until it disappeared when local government was reorganized in 1974. The County Borough was formed by the amalgamation of six former urban authorities and had an area of about 49,000 acres and a population of almost 400,000. Some of the largest iron and steel and chemical complexes in the country are situated around the banks of the estuary of the River Tees. Close to this industrial belt are the old urban centres with a high proportion of poor housing. As one moves away from the river, housing improves, pollution is lessened and the open country becomes more evident particularly towards the southern border of the borough near the North York Moors National Park.

Most health data, indeed most other data are related to administrative areas, and intra-area variation is obscured. We are reminded, however, when national reports on social, educational and environmental problems are produced that people living in inner city areas suffer from multiple deprivations—living in poor housing conditions with high unemployment, poverty and low educational skills. It is important in planning the most effective use of resources to discover if they should be spread in a different way to ensure that those most in need of help do receive it.

The objectives of the study were to identify where the most deprived section of the population lived, to monitor their health and to assess the effect of an improved system of delivery of care.

Methodology

The quality of housing was used as the basis of identifying the inner urban areas.

From knowledge of the Teesside area 20 census enumeration districts were chosen to represent the urban core, 10 to represent the good suburbs and 10 to represent the council estates. For each of these 40 districts a score was constructed based on three housing characteristics, (a) the proportion of homes lacking one or more basic amenities (inside W.C., bath, hot and cold water), (b) the proportion with more than 1·5 persons per room and (c) the proportion which were privately rented. This information was provided by the 1971 census. Two overall scores were then calculated, one of the "downtown" group and another for the other 20 combined.

Having thus found scores for the two types of area, a discriminating value which lay between them was calculated. Each enumeration district in the County Borough was then scored in a similar way, and using the discriminating value districts were put in to one or other of the two categories. From this a map was drawn (Fig. 1) showing the "downtown" zone. (The word "downtown" is used as an abbreviation for the inner urban area.)

The boundaries of the areas classified by discriminant analysis as "downtown" lie along the banks of the river near to the industrial sites. These are the old urban cores of Teesside and include the commercial centres. An extensive slum clearance programme has left open spaces

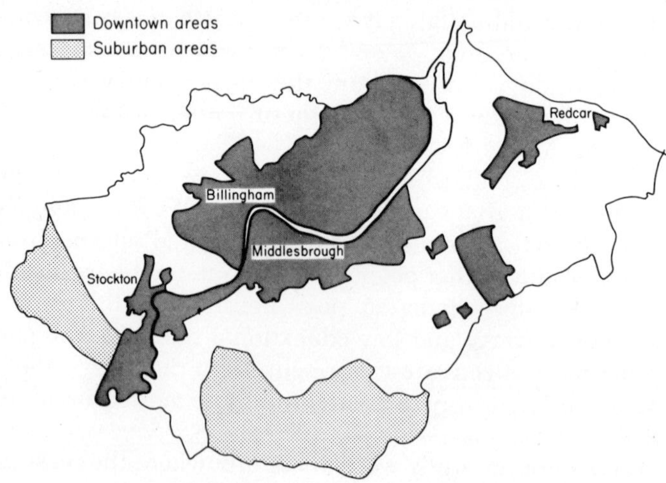

FIG. 1. County Borough of Teesside.

but the remaining houses are densely packed terrace buildings, most of which were built before 1914.

The "rest" of Teesside encompassed a wide variety of housing varying from medium density inter- and post-war local authority housing near to the "downtown" zone to the low density "highly desirable" property in the suburbs.

Data Available

Data were available from four main sources.

1. Census data stored on computer tape.
2. A computerized child health file was created giving date of birth, mother's age and parity, birth weight and congenital malformations.
3. A computer based monitoring system was built up for deaths, tuberculosis and infectious diseases.
4. Approximately 20 ad hoc surveys were carried out in Teesside over a range of problem subjects, from female sterilization to air pollution and health. These surveys were designed so that the data could be analysed to provide intra area comparisons.

Teesside Compared with Other Areas

Data are presented to show how Teesside compared with other conurbations and national statistics for standard mortality ratios, bronchitis and emphysema (Table I), air pollution (Table II) and infant mortality rates (Table III).

TABLE I

Regional variations in infant mortality rates in England and Wales 1970.

Area	Infant mortality rate per 1,000 live births
England and Wales	18·19
Conurbations	
South East Lancashire	22·62
Merseyside	21·77
West Yorkshire	21·51
West Midlands	21·44
TEESSIDE	19·76
Tyneside	19·35
Greater London	17·83
All conurbations	19·97

TABLE II

Regional variations in standard mortality ratios, bronchitis and emphysema

Area	Standard mortality ratio	
	Male	Female
Tyneside	133	135
West Midlands	132	126
Merseyside	127	133
TEESSIDE	120	112
West Yorkshire	118	126
All conurbations	118	124

TABLE III

Regional variations in air pollution, 1971-72

Area	Mean smoke g/m³	Mean SO_2 g/m³
Westminster	58·5	259·7
Chelsea	68·5	234·0
Hackney	70·5	228·5
St Helens	72·0	159·6
TEESSIDE	76·0	94·5
Newcastle-under-Lyme	77·6	122·0
Nottingham	79·1	150·4
Wandsworth	81·5	187·5
Oldham	86·0	135·2
Stoke-on-Trent	119·6	151·0
Salford	128·7	171·5

These tables show that Teesside occupies a median position being near the average of all conurbations for both mortality from bronchitis and emphysema and for infant mortality. In view of Teesside's generally poor reputation for the quality of the air, Table II presents a surprisingly favourable picture.

Intra-Area Differentials

The differences between the inner urban area and the rest of Teesside are dealt with under five headings.

1. Social and Environmental.
2. Fertility.

3. Mortality.
4. Health of Children.
5. General Health.

SOCIAL AND ENVIRONMENTAL DIFFERENCES

Most of the information on Social and Environmental factors was derived from census data obtained in 1966 (10 per cent census) and 1971 (full census).

In 1971, 18 per cent of the population lived in the "downtown" area. This showed a major change in the total population in the central area since 1966 when 26 per cent of the population lived there.

All age bands showed a decrease in population, the greatest in the 0–4 age band (43 per cent) and the smallest in the 5 plus year group (27 per cent). In 1971 12 per cent of the population in the "downtown" zone was over 65 years compared with 9·8 per cent in the rest of Teesside. On the other hand, the 16·6 of the population in the 5–14 year age group was considerably less than the 19·7 per cent in the rest of Teesside.

It is probable that a major factor in this decline of population in the central area was slum clearance, for there appears to be a tendency for older people not to move.

Social Class Stucture

In 1966, 42 per cent of the "downtown" population belonged to social class IV/V as compared with 29 per cent in the rest, and the proportion has changed little since then.

Immigrants

In 1971, 3 per cent of the "downtown" population were born in the New Commonwealth as compared to 0·5 per cent in the rest of Teesside.

Economic Activity

In 1971 the numbers of unemployed expressed as a percentage of the total economically active persons in the area was 9·2 per cent of the "downtown" area, and 5·6 per cent in the rest.

Housing

With the two types of area categorized on the basis of housing characteristics it is interesting to look at these differences in more detail. Overcrowding as measured by the percentage of houses with more than 1·5 persons per room was greater in the "downtown" area than the rest and these differences was more marked in 1971 than in 1966, because of a worsening of the "downtown" situation over the years.

TABLE IV
Percentage of houses with more than 1.5 persons per room

	Downtown	Rest
1966	1·6	1·2
1971	2·6	1·3

TABLE V
Households lacking facilities, expressed as a percentage of total households in each area, 1966 and 1971

Amenity	Per cent lacking exclusive use of running hot water		Per cent lacking exclusive use of fixed bath		Per cent lacking exclusive use of inside W.C.	
Area	1966	1971	1966	1971	1966	1971
Downtown	32·0	23·1	47·6	37·2	69·4	60·9
Rest	3·2	1·3	4·9	2·1	12·4	6·5

Air Pollution

In 1971, the amount of smoke in the "downtown" area was more than three times greater than the rest and for sulphur dioxide almost twice as much. However, encouragement could be taken from the very substantial improvement which had occurred since 1966.

TABLE VI
Seasonally adjusted mean values of smoke and SO_2, 1966 and 1971

Pollutant	Smoke (tons/site yr/mi²)			SO_2 (tons/site yr/mi²)		
Area	1966	1971	Per cent change	1966	1971	Per cent change
Downtown	2404·0	1763·2	29·6	1926·1	1215·1	36·9
Other	766·3	503·3	10·5	847·4	725·1	14·4

FERTILITY

The birth rate in Teesside was regularly higher than the national average, and more detailed analysis shows that within the conurbation the fertility rate in the "downtown" area was twice as high as the rest. It was higher in each age band and was particularly noticeable in the under 20s.

Illegitimacy

The proportion of births which were illegitimate in the "downtown" area was twice that of the rest, the greatest difference being in the 25–29 age group with a five-fold increase. There was a slightly lower proportion of illegitimate births in the "downtown" area in the under 20 age group, and a much lower number of illegitimate births in the over 40s as compared with the rest of Teesside. However, this last age band had a relatively small number of births.

TABLE VII

Total birth rates per 1,000 women, 1971

Age of mother (years)	Downtown rate per 1,000	Rest rate per 1,000	Teesside rate per 1,000
–19	170·4	50·8	70·3
20–24	285·5	174·6	199·2
25–29	178·3	154·4	158·8
30–39	119·3	46·0	56·8
40+	18·8	6·4	8·0
TOTAL	168·4	79·2	94·2

TABLE VIII

Distribution of illegitimate births by mother's age, 1971

Age of mothers (years)	Downtown per cent of total births	Rest per cent of total births	Teesside per cent of total births
–19	21·6	27·3	25·0
20–24	14·1	5·6	8·3
25–29	14·7	2·6	5·1
30–39	11·2	4·5	6·6
40+	3·3	14·7	11·2
TOTAL	15·0	7·4	9·7

MORTALITY

Standard mortality ratios (SMRs) based on the pooled rates for the whole of Teesside were calculated for each zone for each of several major causes of death.

TABLE IX
Standard Mortality Ratios, 1971

Cause of death		Downtown			Rest		
		Expected number of deaths	Observed number of deaths	SMR	Expected number of deaths	Observed number of deaths	SMR
Ischaemic heart disease	M	184	178	97	480	486	101
	F	90	113	125	351	328	93
	T	274	291	106	831	814	99
Other heart disease	M	20	39	195	80	61	76
	F	26	36	138	101	91	90
	T	46	75	163	181	152	84
Cerebro-vascular and circulatory	M	61	95	156	239	205	86
	F	81	111	137	314	284	90
	T	142	206	145	553	489	88
Lung cancer	M	47	51	108	187	183	98
	F	8	14	175	35	29	83
	T	55	65	118	222	212	95
Other cancers	M	53	91	172	221	183	83
	F	66	77	117	272	261	96
	T	119	168	141	493	444	90
Bronchitis and emphysema	M	29	58	200	113	84	74
	F	8	17	213	32	23	72
	T	37	75	203	145	107	74
Other respiratory	M	27	45	167	105	87	83
	F	23	39	169	93	77	83
	T	50	84	168	198	164	83
Suicide, accidents, violence	M	22	52	236	94	64	68
	F	15	29	193	60	46	77
	T	37	81	219	154	110	71
All other causes	M	43	58	135	171	156	91
	F	47	70	148	202	179	89
	T	90	128	142	373	335	90
All causes	M	486	667	137	1,690	1,509	89
	F	364	506	139	1,460	1,318	90
	T	850	1,173	138	3,150	2,827	90

For each of these causes the SMR was greater than unity for the "downtown" area indicating that deaths in this area were higher than the Teesside average. More than twice this average was recorded for bronchitis and emphysema and for suicide accidents and violence.

Infant Mortality

Infant mortality rates are expressed as the number of deaths per 1,000 live births and are conventionally sub-divided into neonatal and post-neonatal, these being respectively deaths in the first four weeks of life and deaths at between four weeks and one year. The infant mortality rate in the "downtown" zone was almost twice that in the rest with differences being shown in both neonatal and post-neonatal rates. With over 90 per cent of births occurring in hospital it might be thought that there would have been a standardizing effect on neonatal rates overcoming the effects of social and environmental conditions, but this was not the case. However, apart for environmental and social conditions there were other factors influencing infant mortality rates, such as illegitimacy. Illegitimate births have a higher mortality rate and there was a higher illegitimacy rate in the "downtown" area with a greater proportion of births in young women. The death rates for infants born to young mothers were noticeably higher than for those in the older age groups, and there was a greater proportion of young mothers in the "downtown" areas.

TABLE X

Infant mortality rates per 1,000 live births (1971)

Area	Neonatal rate	Post-neonatal rate	Infant rate
Downtown	19·4	13·0	32·4
The rest	9·1	7·6	16·7
Teesside	11·3	8·8	20·1

TABLE XI

Infant mortality rates per 1,000 live births by age of mother (1970–71)

Age (years)	Rate (per 1,000)
–20	35·53
20–24	21·53
25–29	12·84
30+	14·58
TOTAL	19·67

COMPARISON OF THE HEALTH OF CHILDREN

Indicators of the health of children and some behavioural patterns of their parents which might have an influence on their childrens health were examined in the two areas studied.

Attendance at Child Health Clinics

Patterns of reasons for attendance at Child Welfare Clinics were studied in 1971 when 472 mothers selected randomly from the 1968, 1969 and 1970 birth registers were questioned. Only one aspect of this survey is reported here dealing with mothers who stated at the time of the the survey they had never attended a clinic with their youngest child. Substantially more mothers in the "downtown" zone were non-attenders, although the facilities were in many cases more convenient.

TABLE XII

Attendance at Child Health Clinics, 1971

Area	Sample	Never No.	Never Per cent
Downtown	100	35	35·0
Rest	372	81	21·8
Teesside	472	116	24·6

Air Pollution and Respiratory Systems in Children

A study of 850 children, a one in three sample of seven-year-olds attending 41 schools throughout Teesside was carried out in 1973 as part of an investigation into the effect of atmospheric pollution on health. This survey showed that seven-year-olds from both sexes living in the "downtown" area were smaller in height and lighter in weight than those from the rest of Teesside. The study also showed that these children had suffered from bronchitis and had been absent from school because of chest trouble more frequently than those in the sample from other parts of Teesside.

TABLE XIII

Height and weight of seven-year-old children, 1973

	Height (cm)		Weight (kg)	
Area	Boy	Girl	Boy	Girl
Downtown	119·76	119·63	22·87	22·65
Other	122·92	122·63	23·86	23·94

TABLE XIV

Percentage of seven-year-olds who had (a) suffered from bronchitis, (b) been absent due to chest trouble 1972–73

	Downtown per cent	Rest per cent
(a) Suffered from bronchitis	9·7	7·7
(b) Absent from school due to chest truoble	13·0	9·8

Measles

Information about infectious disease is obtained from family doctors notification which are often incomplete. It was established that notification patterns were uniform throughout Teesside. The incidence of measles is much higher in the "downtown" area.

TABLE XV

Numbers of cases of measles notified per 1,000 population, 1971

Age (years)	Downtown	Rest
14	11.00	6.700
15	0·02	0·004

Congenital Malformations

The prevalence of congenital malformations was relatively low in the "downtown" area and this to some extent was reflected in the much lower rate of attendance at special schools. It is difficult to explain this change in fortune but it may have been due to the housing policy of giving help to families with handicapped children.

TABLE XVI

Congenital malformations per 1,000 live births, 1971

Downtown rate per 1,000	Rest rate per 1,000
17·81	21·04

TABLE XVII

Children in special schools per 1,000 population, 1973

Age (years)	Sex	Downtown rate per 1,000	Rest rate per 1,000	Teesside rate per 1,000
14	M	0·10	0·36	0·31
	F	0·23	0·39	0·36
	Both	0·16	0·37	0·34
15	M	—	0·03	0·02
	F	—	—	—
	Both	—	0·01	0·01
All ages	M	0·03	0·13	0·11
	F	0·06	0·11	0·10
	Both	0·04	0·12	0·10

Head Infestation

Samples of children of various age groups were examined at the beginning of each term over a period of three years for head infestation. At each inspection schools in the "downtown" area had a higher proportion of pupils with infested heads than elsewhere in Teesside. Furthermore, whilst the levels were very rapidly reduced to a low figure, this reduction was slower and more erratic in the "downtown" area indicating a more intractable problem.

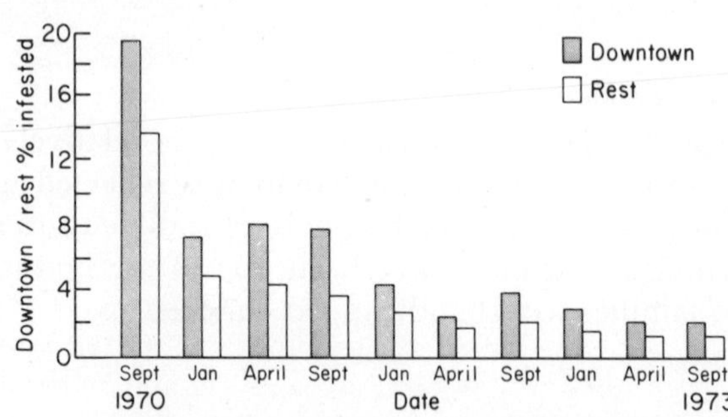

FIG. 2. Head infestation, September 1970–September 1973.

Communications with Health Professionals

One example of the different way in which information was received is taken from a survey of a 100 sterilized women carried out in 1972/3, and designed to study the psychological and social effects of the operation. Respondents were asked whether the possibility of vasectomy had been discussed with them and whether the irreversibility of sterilization had been explained. Table XVIII shows the difference in the two groups. It seems reasonable to assume that the same amount of information about the operation and the possible alternatives were given to all patients yet more women in the "downtown" group feel they received insufficient explanation.

TABLE XVIII

Communication in a survey of sterilized women, 1973

	Downtown	Rest
Per cent who said vasectomy had been discussed	16·7	31·9
Per cent who said irreversibility had *not* been explained	22·2	14·3

GENERAL HEALTH

Some general aspects of health and health behaviour of the adult population were examined.

Smoking Habits

As part of the survey on air pollution and health, enquiries were made of smoking habits of parents of the 850 children involved. Thirty-eight per cent of parents in the "downtown" area were non-smokers compared with 49 per cent in the rest of Teesside. Twenty-one per cent smoked more than 40 cigarettes per day as compared with 12 per cent in the rest of Teesside.

Sickness Absence

At the time of the 1971 census 2·5 per cent of the "downtown" economically active persons were off work because of sickness as compared to 1·5 per cent of the rest.

Deafness and Blindness

Using data from a social services survey carried out on houses reporting the presence of a handicapped person, the prevalence of deafness and blindness was derived. The prevalence of those registered as blind and partially blind were similar in both zones, but there was a lower proportion of deafness in the "downtown" zone (0·33 per 1,000 compared to 0·44).

Tuberculosis

Although tuberculosis was very much less of a problem than it had been in the past the prevalence in Teesside remained relatively high. Over twice as many cases per 1,000 were notified in the "downtown" area as compared with the rest (0·62 compared with 0·27).

What Needs to be Done

The objective of the study was to identify areas of need to plan more effective service; with limited resources it was obviously important that they should be directed to those who would derive the most benefit from them. The problem was tackled by an attempt to improve the delivery of care. It was recognized that just as there are people living in geographically remote areas for whom care facilities are inaccessible, so there are those living in the inner urban area behind social and cultural barriers which leave them just as remote. It was decided to tackle the problem by a mobile task force of three nurses including a health visitor and a family planning nurse, and using a furnished van to visit every house in the area. Six hours in each day were spent in visiting, and on average approximately 200 effective calls were made, dealing with problems referred from all age groups and including immunization which was done on the spot, family planning, meals on wheels, chiropody, cervical cytology and references to other departments such as social security.

The reorganization of health and local government services interrupted this work so it is not possible to give up-to-date results of this intensive effort. However, by the end of 1973 the immunization rate in both the "downtown" areas and the rest of Teesside was the same. Furthermore, mothers from the "downtown" areas of Teesside made up a substantially greater proportion of new attenders at Family Planning Clinics, particularly amongst the younger women.

Unfortunately, the National Health Service is geared to a caring role for those who seek help. The amount of resources of energy devoted to the improvement of health status is small, perhaps because there is so little the NHS can do as social, economic and cultural factors play a dominant role.

This study identified about a fifth of the population living in the inner urban area who are substantially disadvantaged, and it is suggested that data should be arranged so as to highlight areas of need. For too long these inarticulate minorities who need help most have been concealed from scrutiny by the aggregation of health statistics for administrative convenience. The problem will not be solved by pretending it is not there. Society as a whole has a part to play and none of us can be neutrals.

I would like to acknowledge the work of the staff of the Teesside Health Department, and particularly record my gratitude to Mrs P. Birdseye, PhD, whose diligent and painstaking efforts made the whole study possible.

Comparisons in Care of the Disabled

D. M. PRINSLEY

Poole Hospital, Nunthorpe, Middlesbrough, England

The care of the acutely ill or injured patient is seldom a matter of debate, everybody does their best as speedily as possible, within existing financial and medical resources. The care of the chronic sick is, however, frequently governed by policy decisions which may have far reaching effects on standards and on attitudes to rehabilitation in its widest sense. The results can be both positive and negative. Too much money and too readily available institutions can be as effective a deterrent to a return to useful constructive life as limited resources and lack of remedial therapy.

Although hospital resources are very good in Newfoundland for acute medicine, ideas for the care of the elderly are still restricted to some form of institution. After 30 days in hospital patients come under the Ministry of Rehabilitation and require accommodation in "extended care" beds. This results in a mixture of young chronic sick, old people and mental subnormality, all in the same hospital, even in the same ward together with the elderly frail who do not need hospital at all. Planned improvement in provision of suitable hospital facilities still remains behind the times with a failure to appreciate that chronic sick patients require much more than a bed and meals.

It is disappointing to find an almost total absence of community nursing services, sheltered housing, home helps and other supporting services. Here we have an otherwise advanced medical organisation with very inadequate ideas and facilities for the chronic sick.

People are now aware that in the UK there has been a vast development of services of all kinds for geriatric patients. Only 5 per cent of geriatric illness is managed in hospital, 95 per cent is successfully managed in the community by the family doctor and his team of nurses and the network of community services. Admission to a geriatric hospital bed is no longer the end point but only an episode of general management.

Since the Chronically Sick and Disabled Persons Act of 1970, the Morris Act, there has been an enthusiastic development programme of hospital units for the younger disabled, attached to District General Hospitals.

This programme will expand greatly the service provided by existing, often old-fashioned and geographically limited, establishments in this country as well as existing units for special problems such as spastics, epileptics, haemophiliacs and other groups.

Three years experience of one of the earliest of the units for the younger disabled has produced some surprising lessons. The demand for beds is not so great and many of these admitted can be rehabilitated and returned to the community provided resources are available. Adapted housing and a caring family are the first need in this situation. Some very remarkable housing developments for the handicapped can be seen in the UK almost all the result of planning by charities and non-statutory bodies. The Habinteg housing scheme at Moira Close, Tottenham, and the John Groom flats at Finsbury Park are magnificent examples. There is a strong surge of opinion that hospital is the wrong place for both younger and older disabled people and hospital is only necessary for periods of illness requiring the services of nurses and doctors.

There is now a danger that we might over-provide hospital accommodation and institutionalize patients unnecessarily just because a bed is available. Sensible utilization of existing community resources is sometimes a problem in the UK—for example the rigidity of attitudes and spheres of influence in social services and sheltered housing needs to be broken down. Discharges from hospital back to the community may be held up interminably for quite trivial administrative reasons.

Sweden is a rich country, untroubled by lack of provisions for development and seemingly well staffed in every discipline. There are very few old buildings still in use for health purposes. Most hospitals are in very beautiful buildings and accommodation for the elderly within the community is splendid. A typical block of flats for the elderly would incorporate a restaurant with subsidised meals, which also served old people from their own homes in the neighbourhood. Geriatric medicine is still second line treatment and almost all admissions to geriatric hospitals come from other acute hospital wards. Modern geriatric units lack the medical and diagnostic resources to deal with acute problems, although rehabilitation and therapeutic activity is of a very high order indeed, an improvement on the situation in the UK where therapy staff are often critically short. Special hospital units for younger chronic sick patients do not exist and such patients occupy single rooms in the geriatric hospitals and nursing homes. New nursing homes for the elderly are much bigger, up to 150 beds, than we consider appropriate, but by division into smaller units the atmosphere of an institution is avoided.

In Gothenburg there is an interesting concept, a single building housing the administration of all the societies dealing with disability, together with social meeting areas, restaurant, occupational therapy, swimming pool and holiday admission beds. But it is not popular because the disabled apparently do not wish to be all together. Good for them!

The famous Fokus flats for the disabled are superbly well designed but there are problems of isolation of the residents. In some there are problems of alcoholism associated with liberal disability allowances and total lack of stimulus to attempt to have a job.

Much effort is taking place to educate the younger disabled. Placement at home with help, rather than in hospital has been achieved and continued education is freely available but at the end of this process there is little hope of finding employment. Very thorough and thoughtful management of the disabled still leaves most of them at home where "they just sit".

The way of life and the social systems in Denmark closely resemble our own, although the population is much smaller. A policy decision was made that all patients in long stay hospitals must have a room of their own, washroom and lavatory. Modern buildings for the care of the elderly thus have their own in-built problem created by this respect for privacy with many old people deteriorating in mobility and in need of more observation and assistance, shut away from help. It is very nice to see that all long stay residents have their own furniture and bits and pieces around them and, if they have none, furniture is bought for them. There is no sterile institutional atmosphere such as is created in English homes for the aged when bulk purchase of furniture by contract has such a stultifying result.

The retirement benefits for the elderly seem to be more generous. During a recent visit to a city practice in Denmark, a general practitioner had to think hard to find such a case when requested to demonstrate a really neglected old person living at home.

The Danes have a lot of experience in the management of the younger disabled. A purpose-built home—Hoskov Kollegiet at Aarhus has an adjoining light industry, printing, which is attended by residents and disabled people from the surrounding district. Each resident has his own lockable front door, toilet and shower, and no restriction on who stays the night, although the other residents tended to know all about it.

Solbakken—also in Aarhus—has a children's wing and a young adults' section with intensive occupational therapy available, together with a huge work training staff for all types of trade. The children go outside for schooling and many local disabled children are supervised from their own homes. The intention is to educate for discharge into the community. In future children and young adults will be mixed in age groups in the living accommodation so that an approximation of a family group is achieved. The impressively high level of staffing and absence of waiting lists is noteworthy.

The Gjellerup Centre in Aarhus includes special flats for the disabled forming part of a complex of shops, hotel, library, concert hall and restaurant. One resident—a victim of the 1953 polio epidemic, needed total help and had a resident social worker helper, a conscientious objector, doing this work in place of Army Service. Of the 28 flats in this block, 25 residents needed physical assistance. All the residents receive a full pension and extra money to pay for help but, even so, the cost is far less than a Nursing Home.

At Ry there is a special hospital entirely for cases of multiple sclerosis and this no doubt provides special skills in management of incontinence and research opportunities of various kinds but the concept of an enclosed community all suffering from a deteriorating disorder is not a happy one.

Specialization in a unit dealing with a potentially improving situation is much happier. The rehabilitation centre at Hornbaek, which came into being to cope with the polio outbreak of the fifties, now deals mainly with paraplegia cases with great success. The enormous staff of remedial therapists is quite unknown in England.

The Polio Institute in Copenhagen is concerned with work assessment and disabled patients of all kinds, including neurotics, are scientifically measured for work ability. Disabled housewives are included in this assessment scheme in a domestic area and can qualify for a disability pension.

There are lessons to be learned in a big home for disabled younger people in Copenhagen—called Hammarshoj. Two wings are for permanent residents, the third wing is kept specially for holiday admissions. There are many deteriorating cases and deaths take place in the home. There is no hospital contact and only family practitioner care, although there is a big hospital next door. Hammarshoj unwisely publicized its liberal attitude to sex. Although the declared aim is to return residents to normal society, very few achieve this. There is no waiting list, some empty places, and therefore no real pressure to move on. Staffing levels by our standards are very high, as is the cost, about £35 per day.

In Germany, geriatrics is not a recognized speciality and still in its infancy, although enthusiasm is evident.

A national centre for handicapped school children aged over 11 has been in existence at Lichtenau for years. The principles are very sound with children living a college existence with adequate physical help, being transported to a nearby all-ability comprehensive school which has been slightly adapted for wheelchair pupils and where very satisfactory integration of 10 per cent disabled has taken place. The fit pupils give the necessary assistance to the disabled. Staffing of the resident units at Lichtenau is almost wholly by social workers and trainees, who supply not only supervision, but also physical assistance. Disabled pupils going on to University education do very well but the intellectually less able have great difficulty in finding employment. It is interesting to note that the latest resident unit has apparently gone back in development. There are ordinary doors and no washing facilities in the bedrooms. The ordinary doors teach ability to cope in normal surroundings. The bedrooms become sitting rooms by day, clearly better without plumbing in the corner.

In Holland geriatrics is not a recognized speciality and the practice of geriatric medicine, although highly developed in some centres, is carried on in the equivalent of sophisticated nursing homes which are totally separated from District hospitals. Religious orders play an enormous part in long term care. We tend to be too orientated towards treatment and rehabilitation. The Dutch have much to teach us in standards of long term nursing.

A policy decision, a law, in Holland, requires any institution where there are a number of children to have a school. There is a strong special school movement, partly resulting from the consequences of the last war when there were many deprived and handicapped children. Special schools regrettably tend to give rather poor education. There are great difficulties in finding jobs for the less bright handicapped patients.

Deteriorating younger patients are nursed in establishments catering mainly for the elderly. There is no plan for special hospital units. Housing the handicapped in "family houses" takes place where the residents are fit enough to go to sheltered workshops. Grouped dwellings with constantly available help and total privacy are well organized. Het Dorp, a village of 400 flats on the outskirts of Arnhem, has developed on too big a scale and, although ideal in principle, has failed to become really integrated with the town. Nevertheless, there is a huge demand and a waiting time of many years.

Adjoining Het Dorp is the rehabilitation unit Johanna Stichting, where children aged 6–17 undergo very prolonged rehabilitation and schooling all within the establishment. There is now an over supply of rehabilitation facilities for the young in Holland, with resulting retention in such units of patients who cannot really hope to benefit, a gradual change of function because of changed demand.

As in Denmark, the Dutch have liberal and educated views on the sex problems of the young and have actively introduced sex education. Many of the handicapped are woefully ignorant because parents seem to think that disability by itself causes loss of libido. Encouragement of sexual activity is part of the rehabilitation programme and shared rooms are quite accepted.

Future needs have been considered carefully in Sweden and Holland. Smaller family size will produce a small number of handicapped children. Better antenatal care and treatment of neonatal conditions will reduce future disability. Cases of athetosis have already ceased to occur. The Swedes now have compulsory seat belts and calculate a great reduction, in the future, of traumatic paraplegia cases.

In the United Kingdom we have probably got our sums wrong and have plans for too many hospital beds instead of providing suitable houses and flats and services in the community. Present financial constraints fortunately will stop further hospital units being built and allow us to reassess the real needs of the handicapped. Suitable housing and employment is a better objective than bigger and better institutions.

The development of arrangements for the disabled in different countries seems to have taken place against a background of social and financial resources. There are only minimal variations in medical management of long term diseases.

The varying methods of community care already in practice will no doubt demonstrate satisfactory patterns to follow in the future.

Problems and Solutions in Developing Countries

MALCOLM POTTS

Population Services International,
London, England

In developing countries the resources available for health are very limited. They are frequently badly used and the priorities for health care are often misguided. Equally radical criticisms can be made of health care in developed countries and the mistakes in poorer nations can often be traced back to developed countries' over-emphasis on curative medicine, on hospital trained and based physicians and on the use of expensive drugs and procedures.

The Problem

MONEY

There is a relationship between *per capita* income and the money available for health care. In most countries the total health expenditure varies between 3 and 7 per cent of the national income (Table 1), and in many developing countries less than $1 a person a year is spent on all aspects of curative and preventive medicine.

TABLE I

Per capita GNP	Average government health expenditure
Less $100	$0·87
$101–200	$1·42
$201–300	$2·85

This and subsequent Tables are based on World Bank (1975) statistics.

In some developing countries individuals may spend a higher proportion of their personal income on private medicine than occurs in a developed country, such as the UK. For example, in Kenya 50 per cent of the total current health expenditure goes straight from the individual to various forms of private practice (Abel-Smith, 1967), while in the UK only 14 per cent of estimated total health expenditure comes from private payments.

PERSONNEL

A form of Western medical colonialism exists throughout the developing world, with the exception of China, Cuba and the now communist nations of South-East Asia. Physicians have been trained to Western standards, they command approximately the same fees and salaries in nearly all countries, despite giant variations in individual wealth. They are often trained to work in a hospital situation and nearly always with the emphasis on curative rather than preventive care.

Not surprisingly a large number of physicians trained in developing countries eventually come to practise professionally in the West (Table II). One-third of physicians now beginning their career in the USA

TABLE II

	Percentage of new medical graduates who emigrate
Thailand	67
Turkey	22
India	18
Colombia	14

received their education abroad, many in Asia. In 1973 over 7,000 medical immigrants entered the USA. A total of nearly 60,000 American physicians have received their education abroad, nearly 4,000 coming from India, 1,600 from Iran, more than 1,000 from Thailand and 2,000 from South Korea (Mick, 1975). Foreign born medical graduates usually end up practising in areas which native born doctors find least attractive (Dublin, 1974). More Indian doctors practise overseas than work in all the rural health services of that country, which serves 600 million people. A follow-up of 1,553 graduates from the Medical College in Baroda, India (Bhatt *et al.*, 1974) showed that 60 per cent went into urban practice in India, 25 per cent migrated overseas and only 15 per cent went to work in Indian villages. The selection, as well as the training, of the doctors leads to this imbalance and only 12 per cent of students going through the Baroda College had parents with an agricultural background. Among 431 Baroda graduates who went to the USA only seven returned to India and among 65 who went to the UK 16 went back. Two-thirds of the women doctors and one-third of the male doctors had medically qualified marriage partners which is another factor in encouraging urban living or emigration.

A recent economic analysis of the world divided countries into the rich-rich, like USA; the poor-rich, like Britain; the rich-poor, like Iran and the poor-poor, like Bangladesh. A situation is now arising where the poor-rich are feeding doctors to the rich-rich and the poor-poor to all other countries. For example, Iran has just recruited many hundred Pakistani and Filippino doctors to work in its rural health services. Among the many problems this type of transfer involves is one of language. A doctor needs to be able to communicate with his patients, but unfortunately the prestige of a man in a white coat is so great that decision makers are willing to reduce his work to that of a veterinary surgeon unable to talk to his patients.

For obvious reasons the ratio of physicians to population in developing countries is low. Moreover, the few physicians that do exist are concentrated in the urban areas, especially in the capital city, where scope for private practice always exists (Table III). Often populations

TABLE III

	Population/medical doctor	
	Capital city	Remainder of country
Kenya	672	25,600
Thailand	800	25,000
Iran	906	6,220
Ghana	4,207	44,300

are exploding faster than doctors are being trained. Iran needs an extra 1,000 doctors a year to keep pace with population growth, but only train 600 (many of whom emigrate). In Taiwan between 1954 and 1966 the ratio of physicians to population declined from 2,199 to 2,363: 1; the ratio of midwives to people also fell from 5,022 to 5,529:1. The number of people for each local health unit jumped from 2,743 to 3,424. Taiwan, it must be appreciated, was undergoing rapid economic development during these years, but still population growth eroded its achievements.

Not only have limited resources been put into the training of physicians but the balance of support personnel is often very adverse. For example, in Iran there are three times as many doctors as are qualified nurses. In Egypt the situation is no better. In India there is only one trained auxiliary medical worker for every two doctors and in Bangladesh only one for ten (Table IV).

TABLE IV

	Support personnel per physician
Upper Volta	27·7
Ghana	12·8
Sudan	8·2
Yugoslavia	3·0
Iran	1·5
Egypt	1·2
Afganistan	1·0
India	0·6
Pakistan	0·3
Bangladesh	0·1

BUILDINGS

The physical facilities for providing health care are often the least important resource in health care. Vaccination of an injection of penicillin are as easily given in a paddy field as in a tiled, air-conditioned room. Over two-thirds of the world's births still take place at home and a simple, clean room with a screen at the windows to keep the flies out and floors and walls that can be washed suffices for nearly all the surgical procedures likely to be performed at a village level.

Therefore, it is unfortunate that many health programmes, pursued by national ministries and by international agencies have emphasized buildings. It is common to find expensive primary and secondary health centres in rural areas, but uncommon to find them fully staffed and properly equipped.

Western-type hospitals have been built in most capital cities. A famous one exists in Ethiopia where in Addis Ababa a multi-storey hospital stands empty, because when it was completed it was found that it would cost more than the entire health budget of the country to staff it properly. In one African country a single Western-type hospital consumes 25 per cent of the health budget of the total country. In one hospital which the British Government has donated to East Malaysia, the cost of air-conditioning and lighting is equal to a quarter of the money spent nationwide on malaria eradication. There are two intensive care units for coronary thrombosis in the city of Calcutta. One of them is a ten-storey building which also has piped oxygen in every ward, and facilities for cardiac catheterization, aortography and television monitors. There are also two million people in the slums of Calcutta and Howrah with hardly a sewer between them. Cholera occurs quite frequently and smallpox is not unknown. Most of the population is outside any system of medical care. It is a case of diamonds in the cow dung.

Even in desert regions there is a Western desire to build multi-storey buildings, although the architect usually realizes it would be cheaper to build horizontally, often knows about the problems and expense of putting in a lift, and guesses the administrators, who eventually run the hospital, may find it difficult to service the lift adequately. Usually, primary health centres are built of brick and concrete instead of using local materials which are cheaper, more suitable and generally more pleasing.

From the point of view of the consumer of health care a shiny new, Western-type building is often a frightening place. In India the perception of a hospital is somewhere "where you go to die". The villager or slum dweller may be deterred from seeking the help early in the course of a disease and, in the case of preventive medicine and family planning, the cultural barrier can be insurmountable. If the building is culturally acceptable, it is often geographically inaccessible: about half the patients attending a health facility live within one to five miles (Fendall, 1965; Roemer, 1972).

From the point of view of the administrator and decision maker buildings often provide an irresistible temptation for corruption. Some senior politicians and civil servants are eager for international agencies to build health centres, because they get a cut of the price of every bag of cement used.

Priorities in Health Care

PREVENTIVE AND CURATIVE MEDICINE

The profile of diseases in developing countries is significantly different from that in the West. Deaths of infants and children are all too common. Infectious and parasitic diseases often cause up to half of the total deaths in a developing country, whereas they are responsible for less than one in ten in a developed country. Conversely, death from cancer and diseases of the circulatory system are much less common in developing countries.

Data on the incidence and prevalence of disease is often weakest in most remote areas, but a recent survey in Iran shows that in Lorestan mortality under age five reach as high as 34·5 per cent in certain localities. Measles accounts for 32 per cent of all adult and child deaths. The next one-third of all deaths was also due to infectious diseases, such as pneumonia, diphtheria and diarrhoea and vomiting. The killing diseases of the Western world (heart disease, cancer, renal disease) only accounted for one in twenty deaths in rural Lorestan (Arian *et al.*, 1975) The problems of Lorestan are not unique.

Forty to fifty per cent of preschool children in Egypt, Iran and Venezuela got diarrhoea each month (van Zijl, 1966). In Equador in the early 60s the mortality due to measles was 274 times as high as in the USA (Puffer and Serrano, 1973). Further, curative medicine, however sophisticated, is important before such problems. In Columbia premature babies treated in hospital survive as well as in developed countries, but 70 per cent die when they get home (Bryant, 1969). Nearly every case of cholera can be cured in a hospital and while the mortality is virtually zero if you receive professional care within three hours of onset there is a 30 per cent fatality if you must travel or wait for over six hours (Mathen *et al.*, 1971). In Cali, Columbia where the ratio of doctors to population is good (1 in 910) 17 per cent of children who die never saw a doctor, 19 per cent had had attention in the two days prior to death (Bryant, 1969).

FAMILY PLANNING

Death control and birth control must be linked. Birth control faces two problems which do not effect death control: the community takes longer to adopt new practices in the case of birth control than death control and the pattern of investment necessary to achieve results is different. To date family planning programmes have been doctor dominated and clinic orientated and they have concentrated on a limited range of fertility regulation methods chosen for their political acceptability, rather than their cultural appropriateness, their demographic impact or cost effectiveness.

Birth rates, and in particular age specific fertility rates for older women (Ravenholt and Chao, 1975) are falling in many places, but recognized family planning programmes can often take little of the credit. The key factor usually appears to be the availability of contraceptives (and over-the-counter distribution resources are important in much of the world) and the access which the community has to abortion—

whether legal or illegal—and to sterilization. The work of illegal abortionists in India in the fifties and sixties had more impact on the birth rate than all the official family planning work.

Solutions

Despite the horrendous shortage of the resources of money and personnel in developing countries, giant steps forward in health care are possible.

In many countries there is a frustrating correlation between gross national product and life expectancy. Infant mortality, which is a sensitive indicator of wealth, is highest in poor countries (Table V). However it is relatively easy to short circuit the relationship between poverty and mortality. Some countries which are relatively poor, such as Sri Lanka or Cuba, achieve life expectancies which approach that of developed countries (and low infant mortality). By contrast some countries which are modestly rich, such as Iran, still have below average health statistics. What accounts for these differences?

A small financial investment in health care can produce a dramatic and rapid decline in deaths and disease. A few dollars per person, well spent, can halve a high death rate. The most important initial steps in health care can be taken without the immediate involvement of any highly qualified and therefore expensive personnel and do not require substantial investment in buildings, equipment or medicines.

The most important first steps in health are clean water and good lavatories. For example, in the Philippines a *per capita* expenditure of US 15 cents made it possible to build simple toilets, which cut the

TABLE V

Country	GNP ($US)	Life expectancy (years)	Infant mortality (deaths under 1 year/1,000 lb)
Burundi	60	39·0	150
India	110	49·2	139
Egypt	220	50·7	120
Malaysia	400	52·7	83
Panama	820	66·5	34
Japan	2,130	73·3	12
Sri Lanka	100	67·8	50
Iran	450	51·0	160
Cuba	510	72·3	28
USA	5,160	71·3	19

incidence of cholera by 60 per cent. Commonly, there is a relationship between GNP and the percentage of the population with adequate water supplies and reasonable sewerage disposal (Table VI). But it is not a necessary relationship. It is common to find villages using a polluted water supply when piped water could be installed for about $10,000, yet a few hundred miles away in the capital city literally millions of dollars will be spent on running hospital services which serve only a few per cent of the population.

Mass campaigns of vaccination and the eradication of diseases, such as malaria, are also relatively cheap in terms of *per capita* cost. They are nevertheless remarkably effective. Even the inadequate resources given to preventive medicine have changed the face of disease in developing countries, particularly in urban areas. In the middle of the nineteenth century in Europe the cities had higher death rates than the countryside. Excess population from the villages migrated into the towns where it was exposed to increased risk of death. For example, in 1841 the average expectancy of life in England was 40 years whereas in Liverpool and Manchester it was 25 (United Nations, 1973). Today, even in a city as insanitary, disorganized and disastrous as Calcutta the great killing diseases of the past are kept in check.

The investment/return curve for preventive and curative medicine is such that, as medical services develop a stage is reached where large financial investments are made with little, or no demonstrable, return in raised expectation of life. This is the point we have arrived at in Britain and America. The type of hospital and general practice care which we enjoy in the West does little to actually reduce our chance of dying, it is even questionable if it increases the comfort of dying, as so small a proportion (less than one tenth of hospital expenditure)—is spent on geriatric care (Seabourn, 1972).

TABLE VI

	Per capita GNP (US$)	
	Less 100	151–450
Percentage of population with access to water supply		
Rural	13	28
Urban (pipe to home)	21	58
Percentage of population with access to sewage disposal		
Rural (adequate)	7	26
Urban (sewage system)	6	24

The need in many developing countries is to put the limited financial resources available for health care where they will yield the greatest return. Currently, the division of budgets is very similar for rich and poor countries (Table VII) and devotes too much to curative hospital medicine and to the training and deployment of health auxiliaries. For example in Ghana 50 per cent of Government physicians work in the Central Hospital, Accra, but only 7 per cent of patients come from outside the city. The situation is not improving. In Iran, curative services took 50 per cent of the budget in 1966 and 66 per cent in 1969 (Commission, 1974).

TABLE VII

	Health budget per cent GNP	Curative medical services		Public health per cent	Teaching and research per cent
		Inpatient per cent	Outpatient per cent		
Tanzania	1·5	45	50	4	1
UK	4·3	52	44	2	2

The barefoot doctor concept (Horn, 1969) is one of the most valid and urgently needed in the developing world and many people believe it is also applicable to problems in developed countries. In Ethiopia, Venezuela, Tanzania, Iran, Russia and other countries the concept is being or has been successfully developed. A "barefoot doctor" comes from the community he will serve, after a training measured in months rather than years (and covering one-tenth or less of that of a physician) he returns to his community. His work is mainly in preventive medicine, in maternal and child care and in the treatment of common diseases, such as diarrhoea and vomiting in children. A "barefoot doctor" knows nothing of the serum cholesterol or of cobalt units for the treatment of cancer: he or she knows a good deal about stand water pipes and privies, vaccination and dehydration of children. Often he or she knows about the Pill and in China can do a vasectomy or perhaps even an abortion.

Iran is an example of a country currently emphasizing the role of auxiliaries (Rahnema, 1975). In 1972 of $60 million spent on medical training $40 million went on training doctors. Now new programmes of *behvarz* and *behdar* training will change this balance (Commission, 1974). A report to the Shah, by a Commission under the chairmanship of Majid Rahnema, said:

> In the entire country there are 40,000 beds, 75 per cent of which are in Tehran and the other large cities. Thus, the majority of the Iranian population have access to only the primary out-patient services of the 1,000 plus unlinked and generally ill-equipped dispensaries. As a result, while most specialists, doctors, facilities and equipment are concentrated in Tehran and some other large cities, some 18 million Iranians have in practice, no access to the services offered by modern advanced medicine.

In addition to switching resources from doctors to auxiliaries and from hospitals to lavatories a more pragmatic and imaginative approach to private sector medicine could yield valuable returns in developing countries. The dominance of private practice in all non-communist countries has to be accepted. The consumer has confidence in the private practitioner and the traditional healer (Riley and Santhat Sermori, 1974). As has been pointed out people in poor countries often spend a larger percentage of their small disposable income on private health care than a corresponding individual from a developed nation. Currently government services give poor quality, unfeeling care, while the private doctor often exploits patients financially. Is a compromise possible?

The Hospital Corporation of India, under the leadership of Datta Pai, is setting a model for a realistic development of private medicine for the maximum benefit of the population. While government services spend Rs 240 per sterilization, the same operation only costs Rs 53–78 in a private clinic. An efficient concerning service which attracts medical personnel is essential.

In the field of family planning the social rapport which is essential makes the private sector particularly appropriate and the basic simplicity of family planning procedures invites the involvement of the traditional midwife and traditional healer. The International Pregnancy Advisory Services has made capital loans to doctors in developing countries to open fertility regulation clinics. When the loan is paid back, the clinic belongs to the doctor. It is possible to produce services which are very acceptable to the community and yet cost less per item of service than most Government hospital services. It might well be in the interests of Governmental and international agencies to buy into such services, on a case by case basis. They might develop an "intermediate technology" which, at least in the present decade, has much to offer the consumer of health care, as well as the Minister or agency meeting the expenses.

The community based distribution of pills and condoms through village workers in Columbia, Thailand, Brazil and Calcutta has been or is being very successful and continuation rates among users can be better than in developed countries. Programmes run by Population Services International have demonstrated how locally available professional skills, such as advertising, can be successfully used.

So far, the investment/return curve for fertility control has been the mirror image of that for death control. Moderate to high investments appear to have little demographic impact in poor countries while birth rates come down with or without investment in family planning services in developed countries. It presents the politician and administrator with serious problems of priority if they are to make, as logic dictates, relatively high investments in family planning at a stage when death control services are still relatively poorly developed.

If these relationships are to be short circuited then, as in general health care, much greater reliance must be made on simplest possible methods of contraceptive distribution, and auxiliaries entrusted with straightforward surgical procedures such as sterilization, abortion and menstrual regulation. One unit of a doctor's professional time over a year, rationally used and with a humane availability of abortion, could change the birth rate in a city like Calcutta and indeed one illegal abortionist demonstrably reduced the birth rate of the island of Reunion —until he was arrested!

Conclusions

In conclusion, there are gross and, in human terms, indefensible differences in the resources available for health care in rich and poor countries. Some developed countries spend 100 time as much *per capita* as certain developing ones. There is a flow of highly qualified personnel away from areas of greatest need towards those with the greatest wealth.

The tragedy of the contemporary developing world is that planning is often centred on the needs of the already well serviced middle-classes and the modest investment that are being made are going into too high a level of services, which are often inappropriate, sometimes unwanted and commonly just do not work at all. A similar, or even smaller investment, at a more basic village level could transform the health care of hundreds of millions of people in the Third World within a few years, and bring death and disease rates plummeting down.

The money spent on family planning has produced little visible effects on birth rates, while in developed countries birth rates have been falling, often regardless of the money spent on family planning servies. But as in other aspects of health, the inputs in family planning have been too sophisticated. While not minimizing the problem, or the urgency for action, the inequalities between countries could be reduced if there were less emphasis on Western trained physicians, fewer buildings built, and more reliance on the indigenous resources of the people.

References

Abel-Smith, B. (1967). *An International Study of Health Expenditure.* Geneva: World Health Organization.

Arian, A. A., Niazi, J., Potts, D. M. and Bernard R. P. (1975). *Death and Disease in Lorestan.* Iran. (In press.)

Bhatt, R. V., Soni, J. M. and Patel, H. F. (1974). *Study of Medical Graduates from the Medical College, Baroda, India.* (In press.)

Bryant, J. (1969). *Health and the Developing World.* Ithaca, New York: Cornell University Press.

Commission on the Study of Health and Medical Problems (1974). Iran: Imperial Organization for Social Services.

Dublin, T. D. (1974). Foreign physicians: their impact on US health care. *Science* **185,** 407.

Fendall, N. R. E. (1965). Medical planning and training personnel in Kenya. *J. Trop. Med. Hyg.* **68,** 12.

Horn, J. (1969). *Away with All Pests.* London: Monthly Review Press.

Mathen, K. K., Barua, D., Cvjetanovic, B. and Vemura, K. (1971). Costs of treatment and prevention and economic losses due to cholera. In *Strategy of Cholera Control.* Geneva: World Health Organization.

Mick, S. S. (1975). The foreign medical graduate. *Scient. Amer.* **232,** 14.

Puffer, R. P. and Serrano, C. (1973). *Patterns of Mortality in Childhood,* PAHO/WHO Scientific Publication, No. 262. Washington: World Health Organization.

Rahnema, M. (1975). The role of frontline health workers. *WHO Chron.* **29,** 6.

Ravenholt, R. T. and Chao, J. C. (1975). World fertility trends, 1974. *Population Reports.* Series J-2. Washington: George Washington University.

Riley, J. N. and Santhat, S. (1974). *The Variegated Thai Medical System as a Context for Birth Control Services.* Bangkok: Mahidol University Working Paper, 6.

Roemer, M. I. (1972). *Evaluation of Community Health Centres.* Geneva: World Health Organization.

Seabourn, H. W. (1972). Financing the health and personal social services. *Hlth Trends* **4,** 42.

United Nations Department of Economic and Social Affairs (1973). *The Determinants and Consequences of Population Trends: New Summary of Findings on Interaction of Demographic, and Social Factors,* Vol. I, New York: United Nations.

Van Zijl, W. J. (1966). Studies of diarrhoeal diseases in seven countries. *Bull. WHO.* **35,** 249.

World Bank (1975). *Health Sector Policy Paper.* Washington: World Bank.

Health as Aid: The Need for Medical Advisers

PETER J. HUNTINGFORD

The London Hospital, London, England

Historically speaking curative medicine has been exported from the more privileged to less privileged countries as a form of aid. For decades missionaries have been providing medical care in a spirit of dedication and sincerity. However, these opportunities were quite naturally used by the physicians and nurses concerned to propagate their own beliefs. In doing so little regard was taken for the mainstreams of cultural life and social structure. The curative medicine provided was useful to individuals, but without reference to the problems and needs of the population as a whole. The medical services were delivered according to the formulae used in the industrialized countries. The essential unit and focal point of health care was the hospital. The emphasis was placed on the detection and treatment of disease. Later on, former colonial governments provided curative medical services on a similar pattern, but they also began to pay attention to the wider issues of controlling infecious diseases. Such efforts have been maintained and developed on an international basis with the growth of the UN system and in particular of the World Health Organization.

With the distintegration of colonial influence industrialized countries maintained their interest by providing bilateral assistance to the emerging countries. The demand to train nationals in medical skills was recognized; and so, much bilateral assistance given in the form of both expertise and money was donated to the education and training of doctors and nurses. In doing so, of course, the values and attitudes of the donors were preserved and propagated. A process that was made still easier by training of doctors and nurses either entirely (as undergraduates) or for specialist purposes (as postgraduates) in the donor country.

With the development of medical technology the need and demand for equipment and medicaments has exploded, as has also their production and the need to sell them.

Only in the last two decades, however, has the gap between the rich and the poor been acknowledged on a world-wide basis. Only recently has it been recognized that continued socio-economic development depends on narrowing the gap between the privileged and the less privileged. We recognize that the health of a community depends on its socio-economic development, and also that the socio-economic development of a community depends on its state of health. Proper development of both socio-economic status and health can only occur, if they keep pace with each other and are mutually supportive. A consequence of this view is that health status becomes a political issue (used in the original Greek sense of the word).

The medical professions have generally avoided political issues, preferring to withdraw onto the premise that health care is humanitarian and idealistic, should be considered separately from political issues, and should be in a privileged position that makes it immune from the need to compete with other priorities. Some would even say that health and medical care is not even a social issue. The whole of medical training and the privileged place that the medical profession finds in society reinforces such an attitude of paternalism that is still more strengthened by the dependence of the public on the skills of doctors and nurses. Within this attitude there arises a disregard of other needs of society and a lack of willingness to be concerned with meeting priorities. The present arguments about the National Health Service are in my opinion an illustration of this.

Health Needs and Priorities

If we now consider for a moment the international and bilateral assistance that could be given to health care based on needs and priorities, we shall see that much of the assistance that is given still does not fit in with the realities and the political necessities. Still little has been done, or is being done, to deal with the primary problem of malnutrition.

The second major cause of death and ill-health in the underprivileged countries of the world after malnutrition is infection. We continue in our efforts to reduce the death toll from infectious diseases. Smallpox has been eradicated (we hope) from all but one country in the world. Malaria had been reduced as a cause of death only to recur with the decline of the socio-economic conditions of people in South East Asia. Infection spreads because of overcrowding underfed people in unhygienic conditions devoid of clean water supplies. Death rates are highest amongst infants and children under five years of age. To make up for their inevitable losses parents bear more children than they need or want. But it was not until the 1960s that the world really woke up to the problems of uncontrolled fertility. Massive misguided efforts were made to reduce birth rates using the modern technology of birth control. The efforts were misguided because perception of the still unsatisfied needs of individuals was disregarded.

In the meantime physicians continue to cure disease without regard for the consequences, and usually without acknowledging that they have any obligation to do so. Indeed they usually isolate themselves in positions from which they reject any questions that threaten their activities or role. They work in those places where their services are demanded apparently insatiably, and where they can earn a living in accordance with their expectations. This inevitably means the towns, whilst rural areas are neglected.

Curative medicine ensures that children who would formerly have died now survive. Each member receives less of the family's limited food supply than they would have done, the overcrowding and insanitary nature of their surroundings become worse. Because socio-economic development does not keep pace with the rate of population growth social tensions arise from the demand on the over-stretched resources for education, employment and a future in which to live. This is the vicious circle in which we find ourselves today.

Conclusions

1. Health is primarily a social and political issue that must be viewed in the perspective of socio-economic development at national level.
2. Health needs, and the means required to meet them can only be determined at national level.
3. Foreign experts may perceive some of the answers to health problems, but their solution ultimately depends on what can be achieved practically at local level within the limitations of available and limited resources.
4. Advisers should not be used as the conditional strings attached to other assistance. Less would be wasted and more achieved, if what international assistance that is available were to be given on total trust as a blank cheque.
5. Foreign advisers may hinder rather than further progress and development by interfering with the expression of political realities.
6. Inevitably my analysis provokes a negative feeling, but it need not, if having recognized that the promotion of health and the provision of medical advisers are not appropriate modes of providing international assistance, we go on to seek more appropriate ways of narrowing the gaps between those that have and those that do not.

Author Index

Subject Index